PRAISE FOR
Facing Infertility: A Catholic Approach

"The desolation of infertility leaves many Catholic couples feeling alone and misunderstood. Jean weaves psalms, testimonials, and faithful reflections in this much needed book to guide and console those touched by infertility. This book will be a catalyst for hope and healing for many as they discern God's will for their families."

— Jean Golden-Tevald, DO, CFCMC, FCP, family physician,
past President of the American Academy
of Fertility*Care* Professionals

"*Facing Infertility: A Catholic Approach* is a must-read for all who are suffering or know someone who is suffering from infertility. Dimech-Juchniewicz's approach to infertility, a mostly misunderstood condition, is simultaneously deeply compassionate and incredibly informative. She gives the Catholic reader the spiritual, moral, emotional, and medical tools to navigate through the uncertain and scary waters of infertility. I wish it was published when I was first diagnosed with infertility ten years ago."

— Katie Elrod, educator, co-author of
"The Church's Best Kept Secret: Church Teaching
on Infertility Treatment" in *Women, Sex, and the Church:
A Case for Catholic Teaching* (Pauline Books & Media)

Facing Infertility

Facing Infertility

A CATHOLIC APPROACH

By Jean Dimech-Juchniewicz

Foreword by Paul A. Carpentier, MD, CFCMC

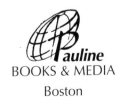

auline
BOOKS & MEDIA

Boston

Nihil Obstat: Reverend Joel Wilson, Censor Librorum

Imprimatur: Most Reverend David M. O'Connell, C.M., Bishop of Trenton
        Granted in Trenton, New Jersey, February 9, 2012

The *Nihil Obstat* and the *Imprimatur* are official declarations that a book or pamphlet is free of doctrinal or moral error. No implication is contained therein that those who have granted either agree with the contents, opinions, or statements expressed.

Library of Congress Cataloging-in-Publication Data

Dimech-Juchniewicz, Jean.
  Facing infertility : a Catholic approach / by Jean Dimech-Juchniewicz ; foreword by Paul Carpentier.
      p. cm.
  ISBN-10: 0-8198-2702-9
  ISBN-13: 978-0-8198-2702-9
  1. Infertility. 2. Infertility--Psychological aspects. 3. Infertility--Religious aspects. I. Title.
  RC889.D564 2012
  616.6'92--dc23

2012009024

Cover design by Rosana Usselmann

Cover photo by istockphoto.com/ ©zoomstudio

Published by Pauline Books & Media, 50 Saint Pauls Avenue, Boston, MA 02130-3491

Printed in the U.S.A.

www.pauline.org

Pauline Books & Media is the publishing house of the Daughters of St. Paul, an international congregation of women religious serving the Church with the communications media.

1 2 3 4 5 6 7 8 9   17 16 15 14 13 12

For John
We entered this desert together,
and you have always embraced me with one arm
and Christ with the other

Contents

Foreword

If you were to visit a foreign city, wouldn't you hope for a tour guide who has lived there and speaks your language? Couples entering the new and challenging world of infertility are like travelers to a distant land. Mrs. Dimech-Juchniewicz has lived in that land, and she speaks the language of a couple struggling with infertility. Furthermore, she brings us the beauties and peace of Catholic wisdom.

Couples who suffer infertility endure waiting, heartbreak, and false promises. They need both physical and spiritual healing. Mrs. Dimech-Juchniewicz has suffered the cruelties, investigated the possible interventions, and endured the difficult experiences of infertility. She has been healed, and she knows how to get there. This wonderful book indicates the path to healing in a gentle, gradual, and sensitive manner. It explains the very successful approach that blends Catholic teachings with the best that medical science has to offer.

The author introduces you to Natural Procreative Technology. This new approach seeks to identify the underlying causes of infertility and conducts research to find the safest and most effective remedies. The primary site of this research is the Pope Paul VI Institute for the Study of Human

Reproduction in Omaha, Nebraska. I was trained there in 1988, and I have been applying their research to couples in New England for the past twenty-three years. The success rates of the Pope Paul VI Institute have been duplicated here and elsewhere around the world.

A study conducted in Ireland has shown that NaPro-TECHNOLOGY healed at least as many if not more couples than artificial reproductive technology centers did, at less cost, and without the tragedy of frozen or discarded embryos.[1] And these results were achieved in a more challenging population than that of a typical IVF center.

The beautiful thing is that these natural methods lead to pregnancies that occur via the loving action of husband and wife, usually one embryo at a time, in a restored and healthy womb, without *ex vivo* techniques. The disorder that was preventing pregnancy is healed, and then the doctors strive to support the newly conceived person from his or her earliest moments.

As a result, the NaProTECHNOLOGY miscarriage rate is profoundly less than that of IVF. According to their own data, on average the IVF centers in the U.S. are losing 6.7 embryos for every baby born. That means they are losing more than six siblings of every child delivered, and that is only counting the embryos transferred to the womb! An unpublished analysis of my data over the same time period revealed that I was losing only 0.07 embryos (unfortunately) for every child that was born. That is a 96-fold difference between IVF losses and NaProTECHNOLOGY losses. Now this is pro-life medical care!

Jean Dimech-Juchniewicz understands all this. She has sought to inform her conscience and studied the wonderful teachings of the Catholic Church. As a woman who has not only suffered the losses of infertility, but has also experienced the joys and concerns of child bearing and of adoption, she is an ideal guide in understanding how the teachings of our Church can help couples, and even the medical system itself, to heal this human tragedy called infertility. These teachings, along with treatment when necessary, can help couples to bring about their heartfelt desires—first of married love and second of achieving a family in a pure and morally licit fashion—the way God intended.

When my teenage son heard that I was reviewing this manuscript, he asked, "What's a manuscript?" I said, "This is the second draft of a new book for couples struggling with fertility problems. The publisher asked me to write the foreword for the book." Then, as only a high school sophomore can, he asked, "What's a foreword?" "It's a brief introduction explaining how cool a book is," I responded.

In a few words, this is a "very cool" and comprehensive book. I've been dreaming of writing such a book for my infertility patients and couples who are not sure where to turn. Still, I'm quite sure that Mrs. Dimech-Juchniewicz has done a much better job than I could have accomplished.

She has responded to God's calling, not only by welcoming and raising her three children, but also by dedicating her time to writing these wonderful words of heartfelt wisdom. That is true stewardship of her gifts.

May God bless your marriage (or your ministry), and I offer deep thanks to Jean Dimech-Juchniewicz and the Daughters of St. Paul for providing this resource to you.

Paul A. Carpentier, MD, CFCMC [2]

Introduction

Blessed are those who trust in the LORD,
*   whose trust is the LORD.*
They shall be like a tree planted by water,
*   sending out its roots by the stream.*
It shall not fear when heat comes,
*   and its leaves shall stay green;*
in the year of drought it is not anxious,
*   and it does not cease to bear fruit.*

JEREMIAH 17:7–8

My mother always said she wanted to have more children. For her, an Italian Catholic woman with five siblings and countless cousins, four children was simply not enough. I grew up with this same desire in my own heart. When the priest who would later witness our marriage asked John and me how many children we wanted, I undershot. I said "at least four" to John's "at most two" so that he wouldn't run out of the room screaming. (I figured God would settle it for us eventually.) I have always wanted as many children as I could possibly afford to feed. I have wished to be many things in life, but my deepest wish was to be a mother. God had engraved that desire on my heart from an early age. I aspired to be the woman described in the beautiful psalm we chose for our wedding liturgy: "Your wife will be like a fruitful vine within your house; your children will be like olive shoots around your table" (Ps 128:3).

This strong desire for children continued to grow on our wedding day. Every time my father held a microphone that day, he mentioned his high hopes for grandchildren. I later learned that a small wager was even going on among the groomsmen. The most generous estimates gave us little more than a year before a child would arrive. Oh, how I wish they had been right!

We started trying to conceive in April 2003. I remember that cycle well. It was the last time for a long while that my husband and I made love without feeling stressed. Soon our most intimate moments were riddled with uncertainty, which later turned to fear, sadness, and doubt. I wondered if there was something we were supposed to do to conceive a child that we did not know about, something that everyone else knew. I would have stood on my head if someone had told me it would help us conceive a baby.

September came. I worked as a Catholic chaplain in campus ministry, and the students arrived full of idealism. None of it rubbed off on me. I was lost in fear. I told no one, not even my mother, of the tests that my gynecologist agreed to begin early, given my mother's history of infertility. My oldest sister Martha accidentally discovered that we were trying to conceive when she spotted a basal temperature chart that I had left out. I was angry that she knew we were having difficulty conceiving, and I refused to discuss it with her. I was in denial. I thought that if I didn't tell anyone, it wasn't happening. In the beginning, I wouldn't even talk to God about it.

The infertility workup was such an isolating experience. I came to hate the purple folder that my doctor gave me with all the information about the tests they were going to do. I hated sitting in the waiting room with all those pregnant women, who—I was certain—knew exactly what was in my embarrassing purple folder. I couldn't even pick up a magazine without being accosted by pictures of bellies and babies. I hated my own body, which was mockingly getting larger month after month, not from pregnancy, but from the binge eating I surrendered to every time my period came.

And of course, I hated my period. The monthly cycle began with a glimmer of hope that grew stronger after ovulation and would build to the powerful light of near certainty toward the end of my cycle, only to be extinguished by the sound of the toilet flushing. It felt like a funeral every month, and I had little time to recover before I had to gather my wits about me and get ready to try again. I was so angry at life. I hated waking up in the morning to the painful reality that was slowly setting in: we might be infertile.

The stress on our marriage became significant. John and I began to bicker, usually about nothing. He didn't think we should worry yet, and I was already terrified. The quarrelling turned into a general atmosphere of short-tempered discord. At times our arguments were so tense they ended with doors slamming and one of us storming off. I began to fear we were irreversibly damaging our friendship.

I had time to be alone only while driving to and from work. My commute used to be my prayer time, but now I avoided talking to God. I had only one thing on my mind, and so far God hadn't granted my request. I went into the chapel at work one day and sat in front of the Blessed Sacrament and said nothing to him. Nothing. I had faith that God was still there. I knew he loved me. I knew he did not cause my infertility. But I also knew that he could fix it if he wanted to. So far he hadn't, and that infuriated me.

The more my husband and I talked about our feelings, the less we argued. After I went to Confession, my pastor told me to set up an appointment with a spiritual director. The more I talked to her, the less I held on to my anger. She brought me directly to Christ, to whom I poured out my sadness. My husband began talking to a priest as well and found it very helpful.

Slowly, our anger gave way to sadness. Instead of silence, I spent my commute in tears. From the depths of my soul, I ached to be pregnant. A test showed that one of my fallopian tubes was closed. Around the same time, my husband's semen analysis came back with bad news: his sperm morphology was off. We scheduled a laparoscopy for me, and an appointment with a urologist for my husband.

Meanwhile, Christmas was coming. Christmas was difficult because I'd thought I would be getting ready to deliver my first child. In the secular world, Christmas is all about children. Parents buy pajamas or ornaments that say "Baby's First Christmas." On Christmas morning they record their children's reactions to the presents under the tree. For those struggling to conceive, Christmas often feels very sad. In the midst of everyone else's festivities, couples may privately mourn the passing of the holiday without a child. For Catholics, Christmas is all about a child—the Christ child. I fought back tears at Mass as I listened to the miraculous story of Jesus's conception and birth. All the manger scenes and Christmas cards made me ask: When would my child rest in his cradle? Where was my miracle? Where was my baby? Why not me, Lord?

I couldn't look in the mirror without feeling like a failure. I felt like I was at war with my body, and losing. I loathed being around pregnant women, but I felt obligated to go to family baby showers. That seemed to be the year everyone else got pregnant. I made it through my cousin's shower only because I was sitting next to my sister Martha and my other cousin, who were also going through infertility. We had our own little private pity party, and we sulked together in envy, bitterness, and resentment.

One day during a meeting at work, a fellow campus minister announced that she was pregnant. After enduring a few painful minutes of feigned happiness and congratulations, thinking no one would make the connection, I excused myself, walked calmly back to my office, closed the door, sat on the floor, and wept. My phone buzzed. Our office manager, a dear friend and a voice of sanity, said she had just heard the news and was on her way up to comfort me. She helped me understand that my feelings were normal, that my colleague had no idea what I was going through, and that if I wanted to secretly dislike her for a while that was fine. But that was the worst part. I didn't dislike her at all. I just hated that she was pregnant and I wasn't. I couldn't stop thinking about my own feelings long enough to be happy for her. My feelings of jealousy made me feel horribly guilty.

Perhaps worse than envy was the guilt I felt for not being able to give my husband a child, and for not being able to give my parents and his parents a grandchild. I had nightmares about losing my parents before I had a baby, and raising a child who would never meet them. I was haunted by the fear that perhaps my in-laws would come to regret that their son had married me instead of someone who could conceive a child with him. I felt like I had to apologize to them and ask their forgiveness. Of course, they didn't feel that way at all. But I did.

My priest co-workers agreed to celebrate the sacrament of Anointing of the Sick before my first laparoscopy. We gathered in the chapel and my husband and I prayed fervently for healing. I knew the theology behind the sacrament. During Jesus's ministry, he cured many people. When he established his Church, he gave the apostles the power and authority to do the same in his name. Their successors, our bishops, along with the priests of the Catholic Church, still share in Christ's healing ministry through this sacrament and the sacrament of Confession. I thought if God was going to heal me, this might be the way. I had clear intentions. I was not interested in what I mistook to be some vague spiritual or emotional healing. I wanted to be physically healed so that I could become pregnant. Sometimes the healing we want isn't the same as the healing we need. So I waited for God's answer.

It came one January morning when I awoke groggy from anesthesia. I'll never forget the look on my doctor's face after that first laparoscopy as she said, "I'm so sorry," and simply shook her head with watery eyes. Even in my half-conscious state, I knew it was bad. God had said no. John was at my bedside trying not to let me see him cry. One of my fallopian tubes was so swollen and twisted from a past infection that it was completely beyond repair. It was removed in a subsequent surgery. The second tube looked like it was taking the same path. She referred me to a reproductive endocrinologist, but offered little hope.

Later, as we sat in the waiting room of our new doctor, I looked around. There were no pregnant women, no pregnancy magazines, and no babies. No one made eye contact. We were all lost in our own worlds of desperate sadness. To pass the time, my husband and I read another patient's discarded printouts from an online IVF forum. The people who posted were hurt and burnt out from the process, which seemed truly dehumanizing and heartbreaking. We quietly agreed it was not for us. Not only did it seem tremendously difficult and expensive, but we were already familiar with the Catholic moral guidelines on the subject and fully accepted them in our hearts.

After he reviewed our medical records, our new fertility doctor called us to his office to pronounce his sentence: "Your uterus is fine . . . IVF will work." With those seven words, our faith was tested in a way that it never has been since. We had just recommitted ourselves to following our consciences, and now we were being told that this one act would surely bring us the child we so desperately wanted. Silence reigned.

Not feeling the need to explain our theological and moral commitments, I finally stuttered, "Um, we're Catholic. We don't want to do IVF. Is there anything else we could do? Can't you try to fix my fallopian tubes? Would you be willing to do Low Tubal Ovum Transfer (LTOT)? We've been told that surgery may correct my husband's sperm morphology."

The look on his face as I mentioned these alternatives told me he thought I was crazy. He seemed to have no interest in actually healing the causes of our infertility. Then came his personal theology: "I know many of my colleagues think they are God, but I don't. I believe that the work I do with IVF is one of the ways God uses to make miracles happen."

This sounded so convincing. He tried to dissuade us from following our faith tradition, and he latched onto a very popular and untrue notion that sounds plausible: "God loves babies and wants everyone to be happy, therefore God must be okay with anything we do to conceive." By the grace of God, we didn't bite. After hearing all about our doctor's personal faith convictions, we eventually made it clear that we didn't agree and wouldn't consider IVF. In response, he told us that we should not expect to conceive a child any other way. If we wanted a family, he clearly told us, we would have to make other plans. We'd never conceive.

It felt like a death sentence. At that moment our world stopped spinning and time stood still. If I knew then what I know now about the miracles of NaProTECHNOLOGY—one of the best-kept secrets in the Catholic Church—our life would have taken a very different path.

Shortly after we accepted our infertile status and began the process to adopt, we received the wonderful news that my sister Mary was pregnant with her first child. I say it was wonderful news, and it truly was. Her son, my nephew and godson, is a blessed addition to our family and I love him deeply. But like a widow whose best friend announces her engagement, I was happy for my sister and sad for me. Her blessing reminded me of my pain. And of course, my natural but self-centered feelings brought guilt. After all, shouldn't I feel nothing but utter joy? How insensitive was I? My sister Mary, in many ways my twin in life, was experiencing what I thought I never would. And I thanked God that we now knew that she would not experience my pain, a pain shared by our oldest sister Martha and my mother. All the women in my family seemed to have been stricken with this plague, and we all drew a deep sigh of relief that Mary alone had escaped it. Yet grief washed over me again.

Throughout Mary's pregnancy I imagined my future son's birthmother. My pregnant sister blessed me with a window into biological motherhood as I awaited my son's arrival.

The next few months brought more and more adoption paperwork and excited anticipation as we waited for news of our son. We had fully accepted the loss of our fertility and mentally moved on. We were thrilled to be adopting. Yet at the end of her pregnancy, when my sister called me on her way to the hospital to tell me her labor had begun, I echoed her joy and excitement, hung up the phone, and fell to my knees and sobbed. I learned then and there that adoption cures childlessness, but it does not cure infertility.

God has an incredible sense of humor. We received our son's referral and traveled to Korea to bring him home in September 2005. It was love at first sight. He was our first baby boy, and he finally made us parents. We couldn't have been more thrilled. While still floating on our new parental bliss, we learned that, against all odds and without consciously trying, I was pregnant. We were stunned!

Our sons are fourteen months apart. The first grew in my heart, and the second grew in my womb. They are the best of friends. My husband and I have had the blessing of becoming parents through both adoption and conception, and we know from experience that neither path is better than the other. They are both wonderful ways to welcome the gift of children into your family.

The realities of motherhood have taught me that suffering never really ends in this life. Though my infertility was apparently lifted for a while, my second son spent the last four months of his time in my womb holding on for dear life. I was in pre-term labor for three months and put on strict bed rest. It seemed like we were rushing to the hospital every week on the brink of miscarriage. Those three months were darker for me and harder on our marriage than infertility ever was, and they were followed by several months of significant depression.

Wanting to avoid the heartache of infertility, and fearing another difficult pregnancy and possible miscarriage if we did conceive, we decided to return to Korea to adopt our third child. In November 2008 we brought home our sweet baby girl. We are truly blessed to have three healthy children, and through the grace of God we have a very happy family.

However, our family still did not feel complete. It felt like someone was missing. After careful prayer and discernment, John and I discovered that God was not done with our family. We began trying to conceive our fourth child in October 2010, and we are back on the emotional roller coaster of infertility. This time, knowing my history and being more informed about NaProTECHNOLOGY, we went directly to a doctor trained in this method. What a different experience! Not only is his bedside manner much more sensitive—he's the first doctor who ever said, "God bless you" after speaking on the phone with me—he actually diagnosed and is treating the underlying causes of my infertility.

This doctor cares about my overall health and is very holistic in his approach. Through careful testing, surgery, and treatment, he is helping me to deal with various medical issues that could prevent conception and a healthy pregnancy. He is trained to be a detective, looking for clues to the underlying causes of infertility where doctors who are not trained in NaProTECHNOLOGY do not look.

My first experience with infertility is a gift because it taught me so many lessons I can draw on now that I am experiencing secondary infertility. In the midst of the ups and downs of every failed cycle, I know now that seeking God's ultimate will for our lives is more important than conceiving a child. I know that if God wants us to adopt again, then he will let us know, and that is what we will do. And if all this time God has had something else in mind and we do not have a fourth child, I know in my heart of hearts that he will allow us to be at peace with that.

I wish there had been a book about infertility written from a Catholic perspective when I was going through infertility the first time. I searched bookstores, Catholic gift shops, and the Internet for some type of support in my spiritual and emotional struggle. The only information I could find was written either by the Vatican or the U.S. Bishops Conference. While this was helpful for me in terms of understanding the Church's moral teachings about the medical treatments and reproductive technologies for infertility, it did not provide the support and comfort I was looking for. Also, even with my graduate degree in Catholic ministry, I found these documents difficult to understand.

So I began to write my story, and it evolved into this book. Through it I hope to become a guide and companion to Catholics who are beginning to suspect the possibility of infertility. Know that you are not alone, that help and support are available, and that your Catholic faith can be a wellspring of emotional stamina as you struggle to build your family. You will discover that help is available from doctors who share your Catholic faith and are at the cutting edge of infertility treatments with effectiveness that rivals if not surpasses IVF. While the pages that follow offer tremendous hope, I cannot guarantee that you will have a biological child. What I can guarantee is that God will remain with you on this journey and that he has a wonderful plan for you that he will reveal in his own time.

I invite you to read this book with an open heart and a prayerful spirit. Each time you enter its pages, you may want to begin with a prayer in order to hear God's voice speak to your heart. Each chapter opens with a passage from Scripture and concludes with a prayer from the Book of Psalms—God's own poetry—so that you can reflect on how God's word relates to your life now. You will hear from many different women who have gone through infertility before you, whose stories will inspire and comfort you, and who will become for you a sisterhood of faith and strength. They have agreed to share their stories in the hopes of bringing some good out of their own experiences of suffering. Sometimes it is difficult for friends and family to know what to say and how to be helpful, so I have included some tips for them if you'd like to suggest that they read this as well.

Finally, I hope the questions at the end of each chapter help open communication between you and your spouse so that you can come to understand one another's experiences more deeply, offer greater support to one another, and allow this experience to strengthen your faith and marriage. God has called you both to this moment to bring about a great work in you. Though it may seem hard to believe, God longs for you more than you long for a child. If you allow his grace to bear fruit in your life through this difficult time, you will come to discover that God's ultimate plan for your life is to draw you closer to himself, where you will find an abiding love and happiness that even a child cannot give.

Chapter 1

Expecting Fruitfulness

Your wife will be like a fruitful vine
  within your house;
your children will be like olive shoots
  around your table.

PSALM 128:3

I always wanted to be a mom. I also wanted my career to be in place before I had children. Once my engineering career was established and my husband and I married, we thought everything else would fall into place. We wanted at least one girl and one boy. However many children we had in order to have one boy and one girl was fine with us, and any extra time it took to build this family would add to our happiness. At least that was our plan.

We started trying to conceive. After a year with no success we got concerned. My ob-gyn recommended going to a fertility specialist to find out why we couldn't conceive. After a few months of testing we were pinned with "unexplained infertility." This was not an answer, and it made the whole process so much more frustrating.

With the help of our fertility specialist, we conceived two times during the next year. Both pregnancies ended in miscarriage. The second miscarriage came with a six-month recovery. Once we hit bottom it seemed like it would take forever to begin to try again, but eventually we did. Every month I just stayed focused on the end result to keep me motivated and to try to stay positive. Each month it got harder and harder to be hopeful, but we had no other choice.

The past three years have been an emotional roller coaster ride. Finally, we conceived and I am now twenty-eight weeks pregnant—well past the point of our previous miscarriages. We've been walking on eggshells since we found out we were pregnant, but every day of this pregnancy has been such a blessing. All of the sadness was worth every second.

— M. C.

Many of us began married life with an exciting honeymoon—perhaps lounging on a Caribbean beach or trekking through Europe. Few of us expected infertility, yet more than one in ten couples will experience this pain and find themselves in this desert.

We may have spent our childhoods pretending to be mommies and daddies to our stuffed animals and dolls. As we reached adolescence, maybe we even began imagining our future children. Perhaps we chose possible names or envisioned future dancers and quarterbacks. As our relationships with our own parents matured, we thought about what kind of parents we wanted to become one day.

Then we became engaged. If we married in the Catholic Church, we agreed to accept children lovingly from God and raise them in our faith. Many of us assumed that we would encounter no difficulties conceiving and delivering healthy children together. After all, we watched many of our family members and friends become parents effortlessly. We then entered one of the most exciting phases of our marriage. Desiring to become parents together, we began the journey anticipating success. Now our imagined future was just within our reach. We could almost taste parenthood. We may even have set aside a room for the baby, began painting, or day-dreamed about wearing the latest maternity clothes. But then, on this brink of excitement and hopefulness, disappointment deals its crushing blow.

Months pass without conception. Or perhaps conception ends in miscarriage. Or maybe there is a child waiting to become an older brother or sister, who does not understand why the wait never seems to end. However it comes, infertility involves a very real loss. Though couples certainly feel this loss on an emotional level, it sometimes can be difficult to pinpoint the source. The journey through infertility can be so infused with "if only" and "maybe" and "just one more cycle" that it may seem like it will never end. We wonder if there will ever be a time to move forward. It is hard to count the coveted goal as a possible loss when we are frantically clutching to hope.

Even in the event of a miscarriage in which a real living person dies, no matter how tiny, many couples struggle with the idea that they truly had become parents to that child. Their uncertainty is not helped when well-meaning but misguided doctors tell them that "it wasn't *really* a baby yet," even though our Catholic faith teaches us that God creates a unique and irreplaceable human life at the moment of conception. Many Catholics who experience miscarriage take solace in their hope that they will meet their children in heaven one day.

Regardless of its underlying medical cause, infertility is perhaps one of the most painful examples of human suffering. Our present inability to conceive a child with our spouse, to maintain a pregnancy, and to deliver a healthy baby cuts to the core of our being. We are created to "be fruitful and multiply." We are built to desire children. We are hard-wired to cooperate with God in the creation of new life. This is simply how God made us. When this does not happen, even if only for a time, it causes us to question our masculinity and femininity, which is at the very center of who we are as human beings. Infertility shakes the foundation of our vocation to marriage and family life. It causes us to question our own identity. If I am not a mother, then who am I? If I am not a father, then who am I?

As a couple moves into the painful experience of being unable to conceive, it can be helpful to identify the sources of their suffering.[1] Infertility takes away many things that other couples take for granted: the sense of control over one's own body; the ability to plan for the future; the capacity to conceive a child with one's spouse; for a woman, the physical, emotional, and social experience of a healthy pregnancy, labor, and delivery, and the ability to nurse her child;[2] for a man, the experience of fathering a child with his wife and journeying with her through pregnancy and labor and delivery; the continuity of family heredity; the opportunity to look into a child's face and see a resemblance to one's own; the cultural trappings of entering parenthood the way most other couples do.

Spouses experience these emotional difficulties differently. Some men or women feel like they are somehow defective in their masculinity or femininity. They may feel like less of a man or less of a woman because they cannot conceive. They may wonder, *what's wrong with me*, and begin to feel like they are the only people they know who struggle with infertility. It can be such a taboo topic that they may not be aware of friends who have endured similar struggles.

A husband may silently fear the end of his family's bloodline more than his wife does, while a wife may yearn for the experience of pregnancy more than her husband. Neither spouse is right or wrong in their emotional reactions, simply different. Infertility also elicits unexpected feelings, like envy and shame, which can bring guilt and anger along with them. All of these feelings, and more, are normal. Spouses should contemplate their feelings individually and discuss each of them together. Identifying which aspects of your experience cause you the most pain will open up the lines of communication. Though it can be difficult to talk about these painful feelings and admit that you may be having trouble conceiving, the sooner you do, the better you will be able to support one another and reach out for the help that is available to you.

Questions for Reflection and Discussion

- ∞ What was your family like when you were growing up? How has this shaped your own desires for your future family?

- ∞ Have you always wanted to be a mother or a father?

Did that desire gradually build through adolescence and young adulthood, or did it come late and fierce? Describe that desire.

∾ What is the future that you hope for? Describe it in detail. How many children do you envision? Girls? Boys? Have you imagined what they might look like? Have you chosen names? What kinds of things do you dream you will do together?

∾ Of all the particular emotional difficulties associated with infertility listed above, which ones resonate the most with you? Why? Are there any other painful aspects of your experience that you can describe?

∾ What would you like to share with your spouse from your reflection?

FOR FRIENDS AND FAMILY

How can you support a loved one who has just shared with you that he or she may be experiencing infertility? First, please pray for the couple. This may help them, but it will also help you grow in your own awareness of and sensitivity to their experience. Try not to ask about their fertility issues every time you talk to them. Wait for them to bring up the topic, and then be a sensitive listener. Let them know you will be thinking about them and praying for them, but that you also want to respect their space. Then wait for them to bring it up again.

PRAYER

Out of the depths I cry to you, O LORD.
  Lord, hear my voice! . . .
I wait for the LORD, my soul waits,
  and in his word I hope.

Psalm 130:1–2, 5[3]

.

Chapter 2

Working Through Denial

Truly the thing that I fear comes upon me,
*   and what I dread befalls me.*
I am not at ease, nor am I quiet;
*   I have no rest; but trouble comes.*

JOB 3:25–26

We already had two children when my husband was diagnosed with testicular cancer and had to have one of his testicles removed. In our focus to get him healthy, we weren't thinking about how his treatment and recovery would affect our fertility. One year after he was cancer free, a test showed he had a low sperm count, which kept getting lower with each subsequent test. My gynecologist recommended that we seek help from a specialist. My first visit with a reproductive endocrinologist was overwhelming, but I felt that our situation wasn't that hard because it was "only my husband."

With a little bit of help we would conceive in no time, right? Well, I was very, very wrong.

After many more tests, we met with the doctor to discuss the results. I will never forget the size of his desk and the view to the parking lot as each part of the awful, life-changing news came out of his mouth. My eyes filled with tears. It wasn't just my husband, it was me! After all these years of being a mom, my ovaries and my body weren't working right anymore. The doctor told us that our odds of conceiving naturally were extremely low and that IVF was our only choice. He also said that my husband and I should be happy with the children we have—as if we weren't grateful for them because we wanted another child. Then he closed my file folder, and it felt like he had stamped CLOSED on it and taken away all hope. I felt so broken, and I left there a mess.

I took some time after that appointment to think things out. I found a new doctor, took new tests, *and* had surgery to remove endometriosis and to make sure my tubes were open and working. We stayed with that doctor for a little over a year, and then switched to our current doctor. This process has pushed my body, heart, family, and faith to limits I could never have imagined. I am blessed to have a strong support group around me, but it is still a very lonely process. I struggle every day with why God would allow this to happen to me, because it's not fair. I am coming to a crossroad in my journey because I feel that I have pushed my body too far, and as I get older it's harder and harder to move on to each new cycle while still feeling such heartache from the one before. It doesn't mean I'm done or that I want to be done. I feel like I don't know any other way than to hope and pray that God blesses us with another baby. I don't know how far I'm supposed to push myself to make this happen, but I know we haven't given up yet.

— S. H.

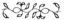

What Desert?

Because infertility involves a monthly cycle of fragile hope and devastating loss, spouses generally do not move through their various emotions in a neat and tidy progression, nor do their journeys always coincide. Often spouses find themselves cycling back and forth through their feelings. Nonetheless, knowing the signposts in the desert—mile markers of sorts—can be helpful. Denial and fear were the first I encountered.

When couples first begin trying to conceive, the mere thought of possible infertility can evoke shocked disbelief. If we contemplated infertility even for a moment, we would begin to imagine our planned-for future crumbling to pieces. We cannot permit this thought to enter our minds, for the consequences of infertility terrify us. We dare not even entertain the possibility. Fear of infertility often leads to denial.

Our denial assures us that nothing bad has really happened. Truly, nothing bad has happened—yet. The problem with infertility is that nothing good has happened either, and we don't know if something good will ever happen. Denial protects us from our fear of losing the future we hope for. Denial puts some time and space between us and the potential loss we fear—an empty womb—setting in. Denial actually prepares us to handle that reality by insulating us from its immensity, if only for a short time.

It might be easy for some of us struggling with infertility to maintain our hope early on, since our doctors are always trying to encourage us, and rightly so. Because we can always look forward to next month, this period of hopefulness can sustain a couple for quite some time. Many people even shy away from the word "infertility," and instead choose the word "fertility" to describe the process they go through when they cannot conceive. They might say, for example, "We are going through fertility right now." This semantic tweaking helps take the edge off their pain and puts a more optimistic spin on the situation. It postpones the need to use the dreaded i-word. However, the only people who are really going through "fertility"—to be brutally honest and faithful to the real meaning of that word—are pregnant people. The rest of us are going through *in*fertility.

Couples who have been trying to conceive for twelve consecutive months without success meet the generally-agreed upon clinical requirements for the category: they are technically infertile. That does not mean they will not conceive in month thirteen, and it certainly does not mean that they can never conceive. It is simply a medical label to describe their current situation. However, most people hear the word infertile and immediately assume it means a couple will never be able to conceive. After all, isn't that what the prefix "in-" means? So infertile must mean not fertile. Since that's what most people assume, it's no wonder that we avoid using the word for as long as possible.

The word infertile, however, only means that a couple has not conceived after a certain amount of time, and that something is very likely medically amiss with either or both spouses' reproductive systems. To address some couples' hesitancy to use this word, some in the medical community have recently come up with a less daunting term, which may actually be more helpful for many people: subfertile. Doesn't that sound better? Subfertile connotes a much different meaning, such as less than fertile, not as fertile as we could be, or challenged in the area of fertility.

This can be a helpful way to think about an infertility diagnosis, because the level of a couples' combined fertility operates on a continuum. This is useful information for a couple to have when they are going through testing. A couple with mild endometriosis is in a very different position than a couple dealing with such issues as low sperm count, poor morphology, ovulatory anomalies, or a shortened luteal phase. However, the second couple might have answers before the first couple, since mild endometriosis can only be confirmed by an invasive procedure that doctors usually leave until the end of diagnostic testing. The outlook for the second couple might seem more daunting, but they may not have to wait as long for their diagnosis. The process unfolds differently for each couple.

Through all of this testing and uncertainty, it is crucial for a couple to cling to hope. It is too early in the process to give up. However, the line between hope and denial can grow blurry. It is one thing to hope to conceive a child in spite of possible obstacles. That hope should always remain alive. It is another matter entirely to deny that any difficulty has arisen. Couples can cautiously move through their denial, face their fears about infertility, and still hold on to their hope for a successful pregnancy.

While denial has its purposes, if couples get stuck in denial, it can short-circuit their emotional journey and lead to month after month of failed attempts to conceive when appropriate medical assistance could have helped. Struggling to conceive a child leaves precious little emotional energy to contemplate anything else. Yet, in the midst of bearing this swirling emotional weight together, a couple who meets disappointment cycle after cycle may also face a host of complicated and confusing medical decisions. The sheer amount of statistics, facts, opinions, guidelines, and recommendations for the diagnosis and treatment of infertility is dizzying. Chapters 3 and 4 will examine and evaluate the ins and outs of various medical treatments for infertility, and shed light on some exciting and highly successful technologies that may be new to you.

Catholic couples struggling with infertility now have many wonderful resources available to them (see Appendix C). As the next two chapters will explain, more and more doctors who share the Catholic faith are trained in a very successful approach called Natural Procreative Technology (NaProTECHNOLOGY). Persistent denial may lead spouses to ignore these options and can also isolate spouses from one another and from family and friends who can offer support and understanding. Additionally, especially for Catholics, resisting the diagnosis can prevent us from pouring out our heartache to God and seeking solace in our faith and in the Church.

Some parishes and dioceses are beginning to offer support groups and outreach ministries designed to help couples bear this heavy burden. If you cannot locate one in your area, contact the family life office in your diocese or ask your pastor or a member of your parish staff for help. If your parish or diocese does not offer any programs, they should be able to

point you to a neighboring parish or diocese that does. Maybe
you can start your own support group, or reach out to other
Catholics online who blog about their experience of infertility. If you have not been to Mass in a while (even if it has been
a *long* while), now is a good time to go back. You may be surprised by the warm welcome you receive. Our Catholic faith
leads us to a well of life-giving water as we thirst in our desert
of infertility.

QUESTIONS FOR REFLECTION AND DISCUSSION

- Have you told friends or family members that you are
  trying to conceive and are experiencing difficulty? If so,
  have they been helpful? Have you told your doctor? If not,
  why not?

- How do you feel about the word infertility? Why?

- Do you think you are experiencing or have experienced
  denial in relation to your attempts to conceive? If so,
  please describe your experience. Do you think it is possible
  for you to admit that there is a problem but still hope for
  a solution?

- Prayer can carry you through your emotional highs and
  lows. God does not expect fancy prayers—just honesty.
  Have you shared your hopes and fears with him? If not,
  why not? Do you think you might want to change this?

- Do you think it would be helpful to pray with your spouse?
  Appendix A offers some sample prayers that you might
  like to use.

- What would you like to share with your spouse from your
  reflection?

FOR FRIENDS AND FAMILY

As couples struggle to conceive, their understanding of their own situation and their emotions about it evolve and change over time. Because of this, at times they may want to talk about it, and at other times they may not. Try to put their needs and desires before your own by being a good listener when they do want to talk, and by respecting their privacy when they do not. Take your cues from them. If they have not used the word infertility, then you should not. If they have not asked you for advice, then do not give it. Try not to allow your own feelings about their struggle to conceive to guide your interactions with them.

PRAYER

Answer me when I call, O God of my right!
You gave me room when I was in distress.
Be gracious to me, and hear my prayer. . . .
But know that the LORD has set apart the faithful
        for himself;
    the LORD hears when I call to him. . . .
    put your trust in the LORD.

                                        Psalm 4:1, 3, 5b

Chapter 3

Understanding Your Options

For surely I know the plans I have for you, says the LORD, *plans for your welfare and not for harm, to give you a future with hope.*

JEREMIAH 29:11

In the beginning of our marriage my husband worked rotating shifts, so it was hard to start a family. After about three years we made an appointment with a fertility specialist and were diagnosed with "unexplained infertility." I didn't understand why we couldn't conceive if nothing was seriously wrong with either of us. Our insurance didn't cover many of the more expensive treatments, so we were told that artificial insemination was our only option.[1] We did that three times. I can remember the first time I was lying on the table thinking that the whole experience was so cold. I felt like a number to the staff. The doctor never looked me in the face, but he just inserted the tube and was done. This was not how a child was supposed to be conceived. How would I ever explain this to my child? But we didn't conceive.

Inside I was an emotional wreck. This was something that I never thought I'd have to deal with. During this time, my best friend and my sister-in-law were expecting. My friend already had two children and had declared bankruptcy, and my sister-in-law had cancer and was supposed to wait. How come they could get pregnant but I couldn't? I'm not the jealous type, but it was hard to be happy for someone else when I felt like I was cracking up inside. Nevertheless, I tried to display a tough exterior.

I was starting to accept that having a child would take time or never even happen, but my husband was determined to find out what was going on. We saw another doctor, who finally did a laparoscopy and cleaned up some adhesions that I never knew I had. The doctor said that if we tried to "just relax"—easier said than done—and if I gained some weight, we might increase our chances. We did artificial insemination with that doctor three times with no success. He suggested we take some time off.

Finally, one day my husband and I were taking a walk and he said, "That's it. No more doctors. I can't take it anymore." Two months later we conceived on our own. We were so shocked. I still can't believe we have our daughter. The entire pregnancy and delivery went without complications. I truly believe that God has a plan and that everything happens in his time. We need to be patient. No matter how hard it is to wait, God's plan will work.

— L. W.

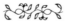

If you suspect that you may be having trouble conceiving, you may want to consider calling a doctor. Something may have physically gone wrong and require a doctor's care. Many doctors will be happy to see a couple before twelve months have passed, especially if there is a family history of infertility, the wife is over the age of thirty-five, or the couple has been intentionally timing intercourse to coincide with the wife's fertile period[2] for six months and still has not conceived.

In deciding whether or not to contact a doctor, first consider that some of the methods used to diagnose and manage infertility raise serious moral, medical, and financial concerns. Many of the high-tech and mega-expensive treatments that have been developed for couples experiencing infertility, such as intracytoplasmic sperm injection (ICSI), and *in vitro* fertilization (IVF), are morally problematic for various reasons. (These and other options will be explained and discussed in the next chapter.)

Further, instead of attempting to heal the underlying causes of infertility, these treatments—collectively referred to as assisted reproductive technology (ART)—either sidestep or override the natural processes that govern a woman's reproductive system to bring about a pregnancy in some other way. Like the reproductive endocrinologist my husband and I saw—hailed as one of the best—most infertility specialists believe that infertility is a disease in itself and that pregnancy (even at all costs) is the cure. But infertility is *not a disease*. Rather, infertility is a *symptom* of any number of underlying diseases or conditions that have caused the reproductive system to malfunction.[3] But all too often, many people are given the diagnosis that is not a diagnosis: unexplained infertility. Others are often given an incomplete or unrefined diagnosis. If you are experiencing difficulty conceiving, you deserve a sound diagnosis from a doctor who will work to provide a cure.

Without an accurate and complete diagnosis, an infertility doctor cannot even begin to treat and ultimately cure the underlying causes of infertility. But instead of healing a woman's reproductive system, infertility treatments often override it or shut it down and restart it by using a concoction of tremendously powerful drugs, the long-term side effects of which have not been adequately studied.[4] For example in IVF, once a woman's reproductive system has been suppressed and restarted, her ovaries are forced to produce an unnatural quantity of eggs, which are then harvested, fertilized in a lab, and transferred to her uterus in hopes of implantation. The amount of drugs involved in this process is staggering. What is not advertised is the risk of Ovarian Hyperstimulation Syndrome (OHSS), which in its severe forms can lead to life-threatening complications. OHSS affects up to ten percent of women who go through IVF.[5] This is just one example of the possible medical dangers you should be aware of in connection with assisted reproductive technologies such as IVF. It can lead to higher rates of conceiving multiple embryos and associated risks during pregnancy. Other risks associated with IVF may include higher rates of ectopic pregnancy, miscarriage, birth defects, premature birth, low birth weight, infant death, long-term disabilities, and increased risk of childhood cancer.[6] You should also know that the long-term health risks for the women who undergo these treatments have not been adequately studied.

Most fertility doctors use these powerful drugs and extraordinary measures because they want to help their patients conceive a child. Like their patients, they want this to happen in the quickest and surest way. They are doing the only things they were trained to do. And the higher their percentage of successful cycles, the higher their patient volume; the higher their patient volume, the higher their profit margin. I do not mean to imply that infertility doctors are only motivated by the bottom line. However, their industry is highly lucrative. The average cost of one IVF cycle is $12,000,[7] and most couples undergo more than one cycle before they conceive. Annual profits in the reproductive technology business are estimated at 1 billion dollars.[8] Of even greater concern is that this industry is largely unregulated by the state and federal governments. As one writer put it, "a woman gets more regulatory oversight when she gets a tattoo than when she gets IVF."[9] In fact, the United States has no federal regulatory agency to oversee the reproductive technology industry.[10]

If you decide to call a doctor, I recommend that you avoid consulting one who would urge you to try ARTs. Instead, consider contacting one who will first diagnose and treat the underlying causes of infertility, and who shares your Catholic values. Appendix C has valuable resources to guide you to a doctor in your area who can help you by using NaProTECHNOLOGY—one of the best-kept secrets in the Catholic Church. Yes, doctors associated with the Catholic Church are on the cutting-edge of infertility diagnosis and treatment. NaProTECHNOLOGY stands for Natural Procreative Technology. It represents a major scientific breakthrough "in monitoring and maintaining a woman's reproductive and gynecological health."[11] In addition to being useful for treating other gynecological disorders, NaProTECHNOLOGY works cooperatively with a woman's body, using, among other things, low doses of fertility medication and highly advanced reparative surgery to restore and maintain reproductive health in an entirely holistic way.[12]

Doctors who use this method will support your faith commitments and have been specially trained in highly effective infertility treatments that the average gynecologist or reproductive endocrinologist may not be aware of. The success rates of their methods match, and in some cases exceed, the widely acclaimed success rates of IVF without the moral, medical, and financial difficulties. In 2009, 47.4 percent of ART cycles in the United States in women under thirty-five resulted in pregnancy.[13] In comparison, recent data has shown that doctors trained in NaProTECHNOLOGY helped up to 70 percent of couples struggling with infertility to conceive a child.[14] Their revolutionary methods are highly successful and in line with our Catholic belief that all human life is sacred. The next chapter contains more specific information about NaProTECHNOLOGY.

Our Catholic faith offers many important principles to consider before making any decisions about doctors and treatments. Infertility is intimately tied to sexuality. As Catholics we believe that sexuality is not simply a matter of biology. Therefore, infertility and its medical treatments have important moral dimensions that fall outside the scope of the medical community. Most doctors will not have any brochures to give you about these spiritual aspects of infertility, nor will they provide you with sound moral counseling. Yet, you must become just as adept at understanding these moral and spiritual issues as you are at understanding the medical information.

What is this vital information? Where can it be found? In order to fully understand how to seek the most appropriate avenue of healing for infertility, we must first deepen our

Catholic understanding of sexuality. Since many of the medical recommendations in this book are contrary to what you might hear from other people, we need to first put it into the context of our Catholic faith's highest aspirations for the gift of our sexuality. For this, we must turn not to medical doctors, but to the Divine Physician—God himself.

Sex in God's Plan

When God created Adam and Eve, he created them for one another. Men and women are made to physically and spiritually complement one another. When Adam saw Eve for the first time, he exclaimed in utter joy, "This at last is bone of my bones and flesh of my flesh." And the author of Genesis continues, "Therefore a man leaves his father and his mother and clings to his wife, and they become one flesh" (Gen 2:23–24). Though Adam enjoyed the intimate company of God his Creator, he still longed for and was not satisfied until he could physically and spiritually join himself to one like himself—a woman. Thus God established marriage as a communion of life and love by which a man and a woman share with one another a sincere gift of self.

Together in marriage, most especially in the loving act where the two become one flesh, men and women reflect the very image of God and his love for all of humanity. Yes, you read that correctly. Our Catholic faith teaches us that *sex is good*—in fact, *sex is holy*—and that it allows men and women to come together in a union that draws them into the loving union of Father, Son, and Holy Spirit in the Blessed Trinity. God created our bodies with a spousal meaning, to be given in a free and total gift of self. While this certainly finds a high point in sexual union, it involves a whole communion of life and love as couples live out each day of their married lives together. A husband makes of himself a gift to his wife every day, as does a wife for her husband. Christ elevated the covenant of marriage to the level of a sacrament, by which the spouses' gift of self draws each person into a deeper relationship with God. In this way the sacrament of marriage becomes a vehicle for God to plant his love more deeply in our souls and sanctify us.

God gave us the gift of our sexuality to draw us closer to him through one another. The act of giving and receiving love during intercourse mirrors God's giving of himself completely over to us, his creatures, in the person of Jesus Christ. "Marriage has God for its Author, and was from the very beginning a kind of foreshadowing of the Incarnation of his Son."[15] This sincere gift of self imbedded in the sexual intimacy of married love reflects Christ's union with the Church as he gave the supreme gift of self when he died on the cross. His death, the gift of his very life for humankind, is the act that brought about our salvation and unites us with him. Because Christ's union with the Church is reflected in the sacrament of marriage,[16] Catholics often refer to Christ as the Bridegroom, to the Church as the Bride of Christ, and to the Mass as the wedding feast of the Lamb.

Sex, then, is of primary importance as far as our Catholic faith is concerned. It is a foretaste of the intimate union with one another and with God that we will enjoy in heaven. Sex makes visible the invisible mystery of God's love, when lived out in the manner God intends. In fact, sex is the act through which the sacrament of Marriage is renewed and strengthened. Coming together as husband and wife, we renew with our bodies the promises we made on our wedding day. With our bodies, we say to each other, "I have come here freely to give myself to you. I will accept children lovingly from God. I promise to be true to you in good times and in bad, in sickness and in health. I will love you and honor you all the days of my life."

Every time we come together with our spouse in the loving embrace of intercourse, we make a sincere gift of self to our spouse and commit ourselves to our wedding vows all over again. Each time we give ourselves physically to our spouse, we are freely and permanently promising ourselves to one another in an intimate communion of life and love that is open to the possibility of new life. These promises are not the Church's creation. They are inscribed on the very act of sex itself, created and designed by God in precisely this way. "God, who is life and love, has inscribed in man and woman the vocation to share in a special way in his mystery of personal communion and in his work as Creator and Father."[17] Our faith merely articulates this truth for us, but it is God's own spectacular invention.

Our sexuality is a gift from God, meant to be enjoyed by husband and wife to renew their love for one another and to work with God to create new life from that love. Our bodies and souls are intimately connected, so much so that what we do with one affects the other. This is why our sexual lives and our faith lives are so closely connected. This is why we should fully understand our faith's teachings about marriage and sexuality before we make any medical decisions to resolve any possible infertility.

Unfortunately, most adult Catholics were never taught any of this—what Christopher West refers to as the *Good News about Sex and Marriage* in his book by that title.[18] It is completely new information for most Catholics, but information that is vital to our decision-making process regarding infertility. In a nutshell, our Catholic faith teaches us that sex is designed for us by God for two main purposes that must never be separated: to bring husband and wife together in an intimate union of persons that seals and strengthens their mutual love for one another (the unitive purpose), and to cooperate with God in bringing forth new life through the procreation of children (the procreative purpose).

These two fruits of marriage, the unitive and the procreative, were inscribed on our human sexuality by God himself from the beginning of human existence. By its very nature, sex communicates a permanent union of life and love through the language of our bodies. It is an outward reflection of this inner reality. In order to come together in the way that God designed, every act of intercourse must be open to both unitive love and procreation. That's simply the way God designed us. When spouses willfully separate these two elements, they are saying something with their bodies that isn't true in their own hearts.

These deeply held beliefs about marriage and sexuality are not very popular in today's society. Many people think of sex as a physically satisfying recreational activity that is completely detached from marriage and from having children. They consider sex to be a private matter governed by subjective personal opinions and feelings. In a misdirected effort to "liberate" sex from the bonds of Christian virtue and somehow elevate its value by making it socially acceptable for everyone—adult or child, married or unmarried, etc.—our society has actually decreased the value of sex and dehumanized it by divorcing it from the deep significance God intends. This has wreaked havoc for women, marriage, the institution of the family, and the value that our society places on human life.[19]

Sadly, these distorted social mores have led to a situation where those who desire to become pregnant are counseled that they have "the right" to conceive and should do so at all costs, and where those who are pregnant and do not wish to be have "the right" to abort their unborn baby. Isn't this painfully ironic? Apparently human life is only valuable when we want it to be. Those of us who beg to differ with the prevailing social opinions about sex are in the minority. Because of this, understanding and following the Church's teachings about the treatment of infertility can be very difficult and unpopular. It can also make us feel very isolated.

Sex in the Desert

Couples struggling to conceive and maintain a healthy pregnancy would love to be able to cooperate with God's plan for sexuality and for the procreation of new life. But because making love with our spouse has not resulted in pregnancy, our sexual love has been unable to fulfill one of the purposes for which God designed it. When we are experiencing infertility, our lovemaking can become fragmented, sometimes solely directed toward procreation without the intention of coming together to seal and strengthen our love for our spouse. Lovemaking can become physically mechanical and emotionally painful, fraught with fear and sadness. We look forward to intercourse because of the possibility of pregnancy, yet we dread intercourse because of the possibility of another failed cycle.

A good friend of mine looks back on her own experience of infertility with bitterness and remembers that she often imagined her husband wearing safety goggles and holding lab beakers. She felt like her most intimate moments with her husband had turned into a science experiment.

Though comical, this image rings sadly true for many of us who are struggling with infertility. In our hope to conceive and maintain a healthy pregnancy, we must never lose sight of our love for our spouse as our spouse, and not turn the other person into a sperm or egg donor in our heart. It's so difficult to maintain this perspective when all we want to do is have a baby.

This exclusive focus on procreation to the detriment of mutual love is one way our lovemaking can go wrong and fall short of God's plan when we are struggling with infertility. Another way is when we try to procreate children outside of the context of our sexual intimacy. In our efforts to seek healing treatment for infertility, many doctors guide us to circumvent sex altogether and procreate a child in some other way, instead of taking the time to actually diagnose, treat, and heal the physical cause(s) of our infertility.

As Catholics, we must keep in mind that we must not separate procreation from sexual intercourse. If we want to follow God's will, we have to do things his way. And his way means keeping procreation and sexual intercourse together. We strongly believe in the dignity of the human person created in the image and likeness of God and in the beauty and holiness of sexual intercourse. As hopeful future parents, our faith asks us to protect our future child's dignity by protecting their right to be conceived and born through our mutual, self-giving love when we come together during intercourse. The immeasurable dignity of the human person means that every child has the right to come into existence in the supremely holy context of married sexual love. Manipulating sperm and egg cells in a lab to conceive a child outside of the sexual love of a husband and a wife treats this child like a product to be obtained rather than as a person with God-given dignity, created in his image and likeness. The incredible suffering of infertility does not put us in any position to alter God's design. Our future children have the right to be conceived in the context of our lovemaking, and we should not waive this right for them. Though we may desire children with all our hearts, and though this desire is good and has been placed in our hearts by God, no one has the *right* to a child. Children are gifts to be received, not rights to be demanded. Just as we cannot demand gifts, because by their very nature they must be freely given, neither can we demand children. As difficult as this is, we may not place our unquenchable desire for a child above God's will.

Inevitably, this means that many forms of fertility treatments and assisted reproductive technology (ART) are morally out of bounds. Believe me, I know how difficult it is to hear this message and to live it out when all we want to do is have a baby. I completely understand the pain of learning that though certain ARTs may bring about the one thing we desire most, they are not moral possibilities. But keep in mind that many highly successful treatments for infertility exist that are in line with our Catholic values. We can choose from many moral options.

Moral Guidelines for the Treatment of Infertility

How can we know which treatments are morally acceptable for us to pursue and which are not? As complex as the medical procedures are, the moral principles involved in making this determination are fairly straightforward. Doctors can diagnose, treat, and ultimately heal infertility in many ways that do not conflict with God's plan for procreation. We can have recourse to these highly successful medical options, as long as we respect three fundamental principles: (1) every human being, even the tiniest human being newly conceived, has the right to live; (2) spouses have the right to become a father and a mother only through each other; and (3) every child has the right to be conceived in the beauty and dignity of the mutual act of self-giving love between her parents.[20]

Let us examine each of these principles in turn. The first principle states that every human being has the right to live. Our Catholic faith recognizes that human life exists from the moment of conception until natural death without qualification. This means that once conception has occurred, whether in the course of natural intercourse or in a petri dish—though the latter procedure is morally problematic as will be explained later—an individual human being is present who must be protected. Their embryonic stage of development does not in any way lessen the value of their life or limit their right to live in a physically safe environment. All human life must be cared for and not intentionally exposed to harm. As hopeful parents, we do not have the ability to waive this right for our children, much less the power to take it away. Because an embryo is incapable of securing and protecting its own right to live, the parents have a great responsibility to protect that right.

The second principle states that a husband and wife have the right to become parents only through each other. We must be careful not to misinterpret this principle as meaning that a husband and wife have an absolute right to become parents. That would mistakenly imply that they have the right to a child, which is not the case, as we have already seen. Children are not rights, possessions, or products; they are people, and they are gifts. Instead, this principle means that if spouses should become parents, they have the right to do so only with each other, not with a third party. The important clause *only through each other* emphasizes this aspect. Because of the sanctity of our marriage vow of fidelity to our spouse, we may not use the sperm, eggs, or surrogacy of another person in order to become a parent or in order to make our spouse a parent. Using these means would violate the commitments we made in our sacrament of Marriage. The dignity of marriage and the procreation of new human life demand that children must be conceived only through their parents' bodies. We may not agree to waive these rights, even if we act out of the good desire to have a child.

Finally, the third principle listed earlier states that every child has the right to be conceived in the beauty and dignity of the mutual act of self-giving love between her parents. This means that children have the right to be conceived in the context of their parents' lovemaking. This is because ". . . *the acts that permit a new human being to come into existence*, in which a man and a woman give themselves to each other, *are a reflection of trinitarian love.*"[21] Married sexual love, a reflection of God's love, allows husband and wife to participate as co-workers in God's own work of creation. Only this context of marital intercourse provides the dignity owed to every human life as it comes into existence. It may seem odd to ascribe rights to a child who does not yet exist, but should a child come into existence through means other than intercourse between her parents, her rights have already been violated. Remember, children are not products or possessions under our control. They are gifts to be cherished and protected. We may not treat them as objects to be dominated from the very first moment of their existence. Children have the right to be the physical living image of their parents' love, "the permanent sign of their conjugal union."[22] Even should that child not come into existence in any other way, we cannot take away her inviolable right to be conceived in the context of her parents' physical union of love.

The defining moral principal is this: fertility treatments that *assist* sex in achieving its natural end of procreation are praiseworthy; fertility treatments that *replace* sex violate Catholic moral principles.[23] Indeed, they are gravely immoral and violate God's design. Because of this, the Catholic Church promotes efforts to research and invest in the prevention and morally sound treatment of infertility.[24]

In practice, the principles outlined earlier (p. 42) generate a list of morally acceptable and unacceptable treatment options for infertility. Instead of thinking of them as lists of "Thou Shall" and "Thou Shall Not," remember that we are trying to follow God's will in the context of the faith of the Church that he gave us through his Son, Jesus Christ. He has come to us in our need in the desert, embraced us in all our sorrow, and promised to never leave us. We seek to follow Jesus as we journey through our infertility. He is guiding us into our future, protecting us, and loving us unconditionally. Following Jesus means doing God's will as Jesus did, no matter where it leads us. If we truly seek to follow Jesus, our guide and friend, he will give us all the grace we need to do God's will, even when it is unfathomably difficult. He will not let us carry our burden alone.

QUESTIONS FOR REFLECTION AND DISCUSSION

∾ How do you feel about our faith's teachings about the holiness of intercourse and how it was designed by God to renew and strengthen your marriage vows?

∾ In God's plan for sexual intimacy, the fruits of mutual love and procreation may never be separated. How do you live this out in your marriage? What effect does/would this have on your attempts to conceive a child?

∾ How has your current struggle to conceive a child affected your sexual relationship with your spouse?

∾ Do you think that your ardent desire for a child can justify any means necessary to conceive? Do you believe you have the right to a child?

∾ Describe your reaction to the following statements:

1. Every human being, even the tiniest human embryo, has the right to live.
2. Spouses have the right to become parents only through each other.
3. Every child has the right to be conceived through sexual intercourse.

∾ What would you like to share with your spouse from your reflection?

FOR FRIENDS AND FAMILY

Couples seeking infertility treatment may be inundated with various medical opinions, statistics, advice, data, tests, procedures, and medication. Managing this and coping with the ensuing emotional exhaustion may feel like a part-time job for many couples. The spiritual and moral struggles that can accompany infertility and treatment create a complicated experience. Unless you have been through infertility, you may feel helpless and unable to offer advice. Your loved ones may also be in a different place than you are in their faith life and may react differently to the Church's moral guidelines than you do. Know that you do not need to offer advice in order to be supportive and compassionate. Unless they ask for your advice, it may be wise not to share it. Instead, offer your continued empathy and persistent prayer. Knowing they can rely on your non-judgmental support will offer tremendous relief and comfort.

PRAYER

Incline your ear, O LORD, and answer me,
for I am poor and needy. . . .
You are my God; be gracious to me, O LORD,
for to you do I cry all day long.
Gladden the soul of your servant,
for to you, O LORD, I lift up my soul.
For you, O LORD, are good and forgiving,
abounding in steadfast love to all who call on you.
Give ear, O LORD, to my prayer;
listen to my cry of supplication.
In the day of my trouble I call on you,
for you will answer me.

Psalm 86:1, 2b–7

Chapter 4

Discerning Treatment

"And now, your relative Elizabeth in her old age has also conceived a son; and this is the sixth month for her who was said to be barren. For nothing will be impossible with God." Then Mary said, "Here am I, the servant of the Lord; let it be with me according to your word." Then the angel departed from her.

LUKE 1:36–38

My fiancé and I attended the mandatory introductory session for the Creighton Model Fertility*Care* System —a method of Natural Family Planning—as part of my parish's Pre-Cana program. At the time I was on the birth control pill to manage my irregular cycles. That presentation stripped the wool away from my eyes and suddenly I could see clearly. I decided to stop the pill and we planned to use the Creighton system in our marriage. But after we got married and began trying to conceive, it didn't happen. Now that I was off the pill, my cycles were anything but normal. The abnormalities had always been there, but the pill had completely masked the signs and symptoms my body was trying to show me for years.

I had learned about NaProTECHNOLOGY at our Pre-Cana program, so I searched online and found a doctor only twenty minutes away who used it. She quickly discovered that I had probably not ovulated at all since I came off the pill and that I had polycystic ovarian syndrome (PCOS). Two of the doctors I saw in college had told me that I had PCOS, but their only solution was the pill. Even as a nineteen-year old, I asked them if being on the pill would affect my future fertility. They all assured me that on the contrary, it would help regulate my body so that when I wanted to start a family, it would be easy to do so. But now I was discovering otherwise.

My NaProTECHNOLOGY doctor gave me a drug to induce ovulation, and for the first time as an adult I ovulated; but still no pregnancy. We scheduled a laparoscopy with a NaProTECHNOLOGY surgeon to check for endometriosis. Instead of just having a typical laparoscopy, the surgeon did laparoscopy with laser removal of stage II endometriosis, a selective hysterosalpingogram, a hysteroscopy and D&C, and an ovarian wedge resection to restore my ovarian function. Four days after my surgery I felt twinges on my left side, saw obviously fertile cervical mucus, and fourteen days later had the most normal period I had seen since I was fourteen years old. I ovulated on my own without medication only four days after the resection.

Since then I've had two more surgeries and have been treated for uterine infection, blood clotting issues, and other immune-related factors of infertility. Most of the doctors I saw outside of NaProTECHNOLOGY respected my intentions to conceive naturally within marriage and according to the teachings of our Catholic faith—but I still had to hear things like, "IVF would be your best chance."

Five years after beginning treatment, I still have not conceived. But the emptiness of my womb is comparable to the fullness of my heart. I have gained so many blessings through this cross of infertility. Around the time of my first surgery I started a blog that helped me speak with other Catholic women going through infertility. Their blogs have answered my prayers in more ways than I could have imagined. My blog continues to help me give a deeper meaning to my cross of infertility and childlessness. I hope that blogging about my own spiritual struggles can help other Catholic women going through infertility. I am also trained to teach the Creighton Model to other couples, and I became an ultrasound technician and perform NaProTECHNOLOGY ultrasounds for two different centers in my state.

I know that God placed this cross in my life for me to use it for good, but the hardest part of this journey is accepting God's will without question. Sometimes I still wonder what it's all for. I try to offer my suffering each and every cycle for other women who struggle with this cross. By embracing my own cross, I try to allow God to use my infertility to strengthen my faith and my marriage, and to help others carry their crosses. Most of all, I try to use fruitfully this time God has given me. I trust that God has made and will continue to make me fruitful in so many more ways than conceiving a child.

— A. S.

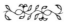

Struggling to conceive a child leaves precious little emotional energy to contemplate anything else. Yet, in the midst of bearing this swirling emotional weight together, a couple who is met with disappointment cycle after cycle may have a host of complicated and confusing medical decisions before them. The sheer amount of statistics, facts, opinions, guidelines, and recommendations for the diagnosis and treatment of infertility is dizzying. In this chapter we will examine and evaluate the ins and outs of all the various medical treatments available for infertility, and shed light on some exciting and highly successful technologies that may be new to you.

Morally Acceptable Medical Options

Let us first examine the morally acceptable medical options for treating infertility. These options can give couples an opportunity to receive the gift of a child from the Creator according to his divine plan. They do not *replace* intercourse. Rather they seek to diagnose, treat, and cure the underlying cause(s) of infertility and thereby *assist* intercourse to result in conception.

Fertility Focused Intercourse

The first step in trying to conceive a child after months of no success is to become aware of the natural signs of fertility in a woman's cycle using Natural Family Planning (NFP). NFP is a way for couples to track the naturally occurring signs and symptoms that accompany a woman's cycle to clearly identify her most fertile time. This information can then be used to time intercourse to either avoid or try to achieve a pregnancy. NFP is a morally acceptable and highly effective alternative to contraception used by many Catholic and non-Catholic couples to postpone pregnancy. And for many couples who have had difficulty in conceiving a child, NFP has helped them. It also gives a woman valuable information about what is going on hormonally in her body throughout her cycle. Charting fertility signs using NFP can save months of testing and can reveal some of the ovulatory and hormonal irregularities that may be responsible for infertility. Charting these signs of fertility gives information far beyond the ovulation predictor kit that you can buy at a pharmacy, and it will prove very helpful if you need to consult a doctor.

At least three main methods of NFP are commonly used: the Sympto-thermal method, the Billings method, and the Creighton method.[1] These methods have revolutionized family planning and eliminated the guesswork and inaccuracies of the calendar rhythm method. All these NFP methods provide highly detailed and individualized information about each month of a woman's cycle. They all involve identifying various primary and secondary signs of fertility, such as internal and external quality, color, consistency, and quantity of cervical mucus; cervical position, firmness, and degree of openness; vulval softness and swelling; bleeding patterns; changes in basal body temperature; ovulatory pain or discomfort; and breast tenderness. A couple can be trained in these methods of NFP to grow in awareness of their own fertility.

Once couples are aware of the natural signs of their fertility, they can time their intercourse for the days of their greatest potential fertility. The different methods couples may choose to become aware of their fertile signs are easily applied if they receive proper training, and the organizations that specialize in training couples in these methods are eager to help couples achieve pregnancy.[2] Couples who carefully note and record all these fertility signs will save time if they need to seek further medical advice, since their records will allow their doctor to evaluate many important factors about the wife's fertility. Couples who engage in fertility-focused intercourse for six months and do not conceive should proceed to further medical evaluations and interventions (and even sooner if there are signs of a medical problem).

General Fertility Evaluation

If you decide to consult a physician, get ready for a crazy, wild ride into the world of reproductive medicine. Know at the outset that you may need to be an advocate for your own medical care. Even if you find a doctor you trust and who will support your moral commitments, you are still a participant in your own reproductive health. The doctor-patient relationship should be a partnership.

Fortunately, many doctors who specialize in the evaluation and treatment of infertility want to abide by the Church's teachings on reproductive medicine. In fact, a Catholic physician, Thomas W. Hilgers, MD, founded a medical institute dedicated to the study of human reproduction: The Pope Paul VI Institute for the Study of Human Reproduction (*www.popepaulvi.com*). This institute is internationally recognized for its outstanding achievements in the field of reproductive medicine. It trains physicians throughout the United States and Canada in NaProTECHNOLOGY in order to evaluate and treat infertility and repeated miscarriage.[3]

When you find a doctor you trust, he or she will listen to you and guide you step-by-step in a morally sound manner. The doctor will perform some tests to determine the possible causes of your infertility, doing the least invasive tests first, then gradually progressing to the most invasive. Lab work should be done to assess the wife's hormone levels, and the doctor might also test for a sexually transmitted disease, such as chlamydia or gonorrhea. These diseases silently ravage a woman's reproductive system and can lead to infertility. These and certain other diagnostic tests are mostly easy to perform, and are generally done, along with a pre-conception evaluation, before starting a treatment plan.

Seminal Fluid Analysis

Though many men are hesitant to submit to testing, a semen analysis can reveal fertility issues that are easy to diagnose and treat. It is often difficult for some men to consider the idea that their reproductive system may have even a minor glitch. However, in general a semen analysis should be done before a couple considers more invasive testing for the wife.

The moral issue involved in seminal fluid collection is that the standard collection method involves masturbation, which presents significant moral problems. Masturbation totally dissociates a husband and wife. It cannot communicate self-giving mutual love, and it is not open to the creation of new life. Also, many men find it dehumanizing and embarrassing. The only morally acceptable place for a man to intentionally ejaculate is in his wife's vagina during intercourse. However, seminal fluid analysis is a necessary and important part of infertility diagnosis and treatment.

The morally acceptable way to collect seminal fluid for testing is by using a perforated seminal fluid collection device during intercourse in the comfort of your own home. It is a sterile, non-spermicidal condom that can be perforated so as to become non-contraceptive. Remember, contraception also presents grave moral harms. The condom must be perforated before intercourse. It can be purchased with a kit that includes a sterile vial for transport to a lab.[4] If your doctor cannot provide you with one, you can contact the Pope Paul VI Institute.[5] You should also contact your lab ahead of time to make them aware of your collection method and to see if they have any specific directions for you. Be sure to keep the sample near body temperature during transport to the lab. Some studies have shown that this method of seminal fluid collection produces a better sample than masturbation.[6]

Post-Coital Test

A post-coital test is done after normal intercourse during the fertile phase of the wife's cycle to assess sperm count and viability in her cervical mucus. During the naturally occurring times in a woman's cycle in which she will not conceive, her vaginal environment is somewhat hostile to sperm. However, on the days leading up to and including ovulation, the wife's cervix normally secretes a mucus discharge that supports sperm health and motility, increasing the likelihood of fertilization. For some women, however, the cervical mucus is either insufficient to support their husband's sperm or can create a hostile environment for it. A post-coital test may also reveal if the wife has developed an immune response to her husband's sperm. Any of these factors may reduce a couple's fertility.

Imaging Techniques

If the tests above generate normal results, couples often may take imaging tests, such as an ultrasound or, to check the fallopian tubes, a hysterosalpingogram. These tests can diagnose structural abnormalities in a woman's reproductive organs that may be causing infertility. Fibroids, cysts, and blocked fallopian tubes are often revealed at this juncture in the evaluation process.

Laparoscopy

If no other causes of infertility are discovered, the last evaluative procedure takes place (although some doctors think it should be done earlier). Laparoscopic surgery often reveals what other tests may not: endometriosis, damaged fallopian tubes, ovarian cysts, pelvic adhesions, etc. Major or minor problems may also be corrected during this diagnostic surgery.

Holistic Therapy

Regardless of the particular cause(s) of infertility, many couples choose to proceed with holistic measures to increase their overall fertility. These measures may complement the standard medical care provided by your practitioner that is described below.

If you smoke, quit. Smoking is known to cause infertility in both men and women.[7] Smoking also makes it more difficult to carry a pregnancy to term. Additionally, twelve percent of infertility cases can be linked to a woman either weighing too much or too little.[8] This is because estrogen, a necessary hormonal ingredient for fertility, is produced in fat cells. Having too much or too little body fat may negatively affect a woman's estrogen levels. Further, researchers have found a relationship between fat consumption and semen quality in men. The more saturated and monounsaturated fats a man consumes, the lower his sperm count. However, polyunsaturated fat intake seems to have beneficial effects on fertility.[9]

Not smoking and weight management are not only important for overall health for both men and women, but they are also important for fertility.

Many people wonder if there is a connection between nutrition, vitamin supplements, and fertility. While it is well-known that a healthy diet high in vitamins and minerals contributes to overall health, little is known about any particular correlations with reproductive health. However, many women and NaProTECHNOLOGY doctors have successfully achieved increases in cervical mucus using natural enhancers such as vitamin B6 and guaifenesin (an expectorant found in some over the counter cough syrups). While this is certainly an off-label use, under a doctor's supervision they have been shown to be helpful for many women with scanty cervical mucus. Amoxicillin can also be used for this purpose.[10]

Finally, a word about stress. If you haven't heard it yet, you probably will: "Just relax and you'll get pregnant!" That's infuriating and untrue. There is absolutely no proof that underlying stress causes or in any way contributes to infertility.[11] On the other hand, it is an understatement to say that infertility causes stress. Infertility causes *tremendous* stress. Many men and women seek out stress management techniques as they go through infertility simply to relieve some of the burden they carry. My husband and I found prayer extremely helpful, and we prayed alone and together. We especially took solace in the comforting words of the psalms that are included in Night Prayer from the Liturgy of the Hours, and in the prayer to Saint Gerard.[12] My husband also developed a significant devotion to Saint Joseph and began praying the Rosary. I know many women who journeyed through infertility with a purse full of prayer cards, holy pictures, and medals of various saints. John and

I found it helpful to frequent the sacraments and relied upon our priests and spiritual directors for support. I also found myself sitting in front of the Blessed Sacrament in silence more and more often. Prayer is a source of peace and strength, which also tends to relieve stress. But other methods of reducing stress may appeal to you as well. Many couples try relaxation, meditation, acupuncture, and the like to reduce the stress that comes along with fertility evaluation and treatment.

Fertility Drug Therapy

If a hormonal imbalance or deficiency is identified, or if an infection is present, hormone supplementation or drug therapy may correct the problem. The fertility of both husband and wife can often be enhanced by hormone therapy.

Reparative Surgery

When structural abnormality or damage is present, surgery is usually required to correct the condition. Most urologists can easily treat varicoceles[13] and specialized gynecologists can remove endometriosis, cysts, polyps, and fibroids. Yet, a highly-skilled reproductive surgeon might be the best one to remove even the tiniest spot of endometriosis, to delicately open blocked fallopian tubes, and to remove damaged portions of fallopian tubes and reattach the healthy portions. However, it is difficult to find a reproductive surgeon who is capable of successfully performing all of these very delicate surgical procedures.

That is because when IVF became available after 1978, reproductive medicine shifted gears. Fewer doctors were trained to perform restorative reproductive surgery, and more doctors were trained to override women's reproductive systems and replace sexual intercourse with a lab procedure through IVF. Therefore, most reproductive specialists will not attempt to do the kinds of things that need to be done in order to restore reproductive health. They simply were never trained to do so.[14]

Fortunately, because the Pope Paul VI Institute for the Study of Human Reproduction is aligned with the Catholic Church's moral teachings regarding the treatment of infertility, restorative reproductive surgery has continued to advance in the United States and Canada. Doctors who are fellowship trained by the Pope Paul VI Institute are advanced specialists in a highly-skilled area of surgical techniques that can actually structurally rebuild and restore reproductive health in ways other reproductive endocrinologists cannot. They are also very skilled in reproductive medicine. The Institute also has a certificate program for various aspects of procreative medicine for non-surgical doctors and nurse practitioners.

I didn't know about the Pope Paul VI Institute when my husband and I were going through our infertility. My reproductive endocrinologist had never heard of it either. That is why he thought I was crazy when I asked him if he could repair my fallopian tubes. Instead, he removed one. To his credit, however, he knew our position on IVF and forced the weakest trickle of dye through my remaining fallopian tube during surgery. Because it was so twisted and scarred, he warned me that it would probably close within a week. We hadn't even scheduled my husband's surgery for bilateral varicoceles, yet we were assured that we had no chance of ever conceiving.

A year and a half later, in the midst of adopting our oldest son from Korea, our second son was inexplicably conceived. My husband's surgery must have worked, and my remaining fallopian tube, damaged and scarred as it was, must have still been open after all that time. Two by two, God sent us the most precious sons we could ever have hoped for. The first began to grow in my heart as soon as I received his referral photo, and, unbeknownst to us, the second began to grow several months later under my heart, right next to his brother.

Low Tubal Ovum Transfer (LTOT)

If tubal function cannot be restored through surgery, a procedure known as Low Tubal Ovum Transfer (LTOT) can be performed. In LTOT, a woman's ovum is transferred below the point of tubal damage or blockage, or sometimes within the uterus, prior to normal intercourse during the fertile phase of her cycle. Most theologians consider this treatment to be morally acceptable.[15]

LTOT and the other preceding medical treatment options for infertility are just that—treatments. I would like to stress again that the key to successfully treating infertility and restoring reproductive health is diagnosing the underlying disorder(s) causing infertility. Infertility is not a *disease*; it is a *symptom* of an underlying medical condition. It is a physical limitation that is caused by a physical disorder. Even in cases of "unexplained infertility," something has physically gone wrong. There is always an underlying disorder, even when its nature cannot be determined. The goal of these tests and treatments is to diagnose, treat, and ultimately cure the underlying cause of infertility. They are meant to assist intercourse, not replace it, in conceiving a child.

Morally Unacceptable Medical Options

Now that we have explored all of the morally acceptable medical treatments, let us see why others are not morally acceptable.[16] Though these procedures may seem to be treatments for infertility, they are really replacements for sexual intimacy that bypass the causes of infertility and conceive children outside the sexual union of marital love. "The replacement of the conjugal act by a technical procedure . . . leads to a weakening of the respect owed to every human being,"[17] and for this reason is determined to be morally unacceptable.

Obtaining Semen Through Masturbation

Whenever donor sperm is used, and frequently when a husband's sperm is used, it is collected through masturbation. This is immoral for all of the reasons described above in the section on Seminal Fluid Analysis. Masturbation is never a morally acceptable means to obtain sperm, whether it is for analysis of male factor infertility or for use in ART. The ends do not justify the means. A couple should instead use a perforated seminal fluid collection device to generate a sample.

Heterologous Procedures

These are procedures in which a third party is used to bring about conception through the use of donor sperm, donor eggs, or both donor sperm and eggs. Heterologous procedures also include surrogacy, in which another woman is impregnated with a fertilized egg and gestates a child for an infertile couple. Donor and couple gametes are often used in different combinations and in various procedures, such as artificial insemination, intrauterine injection, intracytoplasmic sperm injection, *in vitro* fertilization, and surrogacy. No matter which procedure is used, all heterologous procedures are considered gravely immoral. First, they violate the rights of the husband and wife to become father and mother only through each other, and as such breach the marriage vow of fidelity. Second, many of these procedures separate procreation from lovemaking, violating the child's right to be conceived in the beauty and dignity of the parents' act of self-giving love in intercourse. Finally, the donor sperm is most often collected through masturbation, which is not morally acceptable.[18]

Zygote Intrafallopian Transfer (ZIFT)

In this procedure, a sperm and egg are combined outside the wife's body, and the zygote (newly fertilized embryo) is transferred to her fallopian tube. This is done to bypass, rather than treat, a number of fertility problems. Even if the husband's sperm was collected in a morally acceptable way, this procedure still replaces sexual intercourse and separates it from procreation because conception takes place outside of the wife's body. Thus, it deprives the child of his right to be conceived in the context of his parent's lovemaking, making the child an object to be manipulated rather than a gift to be received.

Intracytoplasmic Sperm Injection (ICSI)

In this procedure, a single sperm is injected directly into the ovum to bypass certain forms of male factor infertility. The resulting embryo is then transferred into the woman's body for implantation. Like ZIFT, even if the husband's sperm was collected in a morally acceptable way, this procedure still replaces sexual intercourse and separates it from procreation because conception takes place outside the wife's body. It causes "a complete separation between procreation and the conjugal act."[19] Thus, it deprives the child of his right to be conceived in the context of his parent's lovemaking.

In Vitro Fertilization (IVF)

IVF is now one of the most common forms of ART. It involves the artificial conception of human life through the fertilization of ova from the wife or a donor by sperm from the husband or a donor. Generally speaking, a large number of embryos are created in a petri dish and observed for growth. A certain number are then transferred to the uterus of the wife or a surrogate in hopes of implantation. A certain number of embryos may also be frozen for future use, and a certain number may be destroyed because they are found to be "defective."

We've already considered the moral problems involved when a third party (egg donor, sperm donor, or surrogate) is introduced to bring about procreation. These types of procedures deprive the husband and wife of their right to become a parent only through each other. We've also considered the immorality of the collection of sperm through masturbation. So let's consider a hypothetical (and rare) case in which the couple does not use donor gametes and even collects a semen sample with a perforated condom, thus bypassing certain moral problems. IVF still necessarily involves the creation of human life in a petri dish. IVF always dissociates procreation from the sexual union of the spouses, thus depriving the embryos of their basic human right to be conceived in the dignity of their parents' act of mutual love. These tiny embryos, children of the husband and wife, "are human beings and subjects with rights: their dignity and right to life must be respected from the first moment of their existence."[20]

Usually at least two or more embryos are transferred for implantation. The others are then exposed to an absurd fate. These tiny pre-born children are either discarded or frozen. Discarding human life is, of course, morally reprehensible. Freezing human embryos, "even when carried out in order to preserve the life of an embryo—cryopreservation—*constitutes an offense against the respect due to human beings* by exposing them to grave risks of death or harm to their physical integrity and depriving them, at least temporarily, of maternal shelter and gestation, thus placing them in a situation in which further offenses and manipulation are possible."[21] Further, "the majority of embryos that are not used remain 'orphans.' Their parents do not ask for them and at times all trace of the parents is lost. This is why there are thousands upon thousands of frozen embryos in almost all countries where *in vitro* fertilization takes place."[22]

So let's consider a case in which all of the embryos were transferred for implantation and none were frozen. If the doctor determines that too great a number of embryos implant successfully, the couple is usually then asked to reduce the number of embryos through selective abortion, which is, of course, like all procured abortion, gravely immoral. Even if the couple implants all the embryos they have fertilized and do not selectively abort any that survive, IVF is still gravely morally wrong. It totally dissociates procreation from the act of self-giving love of marital intercourse, depriving the children conceived of a basic human right.

Along with ZIFT and ICSI, IVF devalues the human person and treats tiny human beings as if they are mere biological material to be manipulated or thrown away. Further, and perhaps even more disturbing, "cases are becoming ever more prevalent in which couples who have no fertility problems are using artificial means of procreation in order to engage in genetic selection of their offspring."[23] This practice puts a doctor in the place of the Divine Physician and leaves no creative artistry in God's hands.

Human Cloning

In human cloning, the nucleus of a body cell is transferred into an egg cell to produce a new human being who is an identical genetic copy of the donor of the body cell. Though not currently used in fertility treatments, human cloning is proposed as a way for infertile couples to have a baby. The possibility of cloning a copy of a human being has given rise to serious concern throughout the world, and is prohibited in many nations. It reduces human reproduction to a manufacturing process and treats the human embryo as a thing or commodity, a mere copy of someone else. It is not connected to human sexuality at all, indeed it is *asexual*: it does not require the use of a potential father's sperm. "Human cloning is intrinsically illicit in that, by taking the ethical negativity of techniques of artificial fertilization to their extreme, it seeks to *give rise to a new human being without a connection to the act of reciprocal self-giving between the spouses* and, more radically, *without any link to sexuality*. This leads to manipulation and abuses gravely injurious to human dignity."[24] Human cloning represents one of the grossest violations of human dignity ever made possible by medical research.[25]

Medical Options Currently under Discussion (Neither "Approved" nor "Disapproved")

In addition to the tests and treatments listed above, some medical procedures and treatments fall into a gray area because they are currently under discussion among Church authorities. The Church has not declared them to be either moral or immoral.

As you will see, a moral determination on these procedures is difficult because it can be considered unclear whether or not these procedures *assist* sexual intercourse in achieving its natural end or if they *replace* intercourse altogether. Even highly educated Catholic theologians respectfully disagree about the morality of these options. Since there has been no official definitive decision either for or against these procedures, Catholics should approach these with great caution and carefully form their consciences with faithfulness to the moral guidelines set forth by the Church. It is recommended that couples discuss these options with a priest who will help them carefully consider their situation in light of the Church's moral guidelines for discerning treatment.

Gamete Intra-Fallopian Transfer (GIFT)

In this procedure, the wife's ovum is surgically removed from her body and placed in a catheter, along with morally-obtained (non-masturbatory) sperm from her husband from a previous act of intercourse with a perforated condom. The ovum and sperm are separated by an air-bubble in the catheter and injected into the wife's uterus, where fertilization can occur. This procedure can take place either before or after normal intercourse. Catholic theologians disagree about the morality of this procedure. Some believe that it assists normal intercourse in achieving procreation, while others argue that it replaces intercourse.[26]

Tubal Ovum Transfer with Sperm (TOTS)

This procedure is very similar to GIFT. The egg and sperm are collected in a morally acceptable way and placed in a catheter separated by an air bubble. Instead of injecting them into the wife's uterus, they are injected into her fallopian tube, where fertilization can occur. For the same reasons as with GIFT, Catholic moral theologians disagree about the morality of this procedure, so couples are free to seek this medical option if their own consciences permit.

Intra-Uterine Insemination (IUI) with Husband's Morally-Obtained Sperm

This procedure is only considered "under discussion" when it uses the husband's sperm, and when this sperm has been obtained through normal intercourse with a perforated condom. (The use of donor sperm for IUI, or even the husband's sperm when obtained through masturbation, is always considered immoral for reasons discussed earlier.) After normal intercourse, the remaining sperm is collected from the perforated condom and injected directly into the wife's uterus, bypassing the cervix and a potentially hostile vaginal environment, in the hopes that fertilization will occur. This procedure can be used to treat conditions of infertility in which the husband's sperm does not survive until it can fertilize the wife's ovum, or in which structural abnormalities prevent the passage of sperm into the wife's uterus. This procedure can be admitted "for those cases in which the technical means is not a substitute for the conjugal act but serves to facilitate and to help so that the act attains its natural purpose."[27]

Embryo Adoption

As of 2002, there were nearly 400,000 human embryos frozen in storage facilities at fertility clinics throughout the United States.[28] And the number of frozen embryos in Canada is unknown.[29] There is no more recent data available because fertility clinics are notoriously under-regulated. They do not have to report when embryos are created, placed into or taken out of storage, or what is done with them. But every year since 2002, fertility clinics throughout the United States have reportedly performed well over 100,000 cycles of assisted reproductive technology, with these numbers steadily increasing. The number of embryos produced is rising, while the number of embryos transferred in a given cycle is decreasing to lessen the likelihood of multiple births.[30] These tiny human beings, frozen indefinitely, are the byproducts of a largely unregulated fertility industry. Surely their staggering numbers have grown substantially over the years.

This situation raises a serious moral dilemma about the fate of these frozen embryos. What, if any, moral options are available to give these little frozen human beings a chance at survival? It would be seriously wrong to produce embryos through *in vitro* fertilization for the express purpose of donating them to other couples as a treatment for infertility. However, since these tiny human beings already exist through no direct action of the prospective adoptive parents, many Catholic bioethicists and moral theologians have asked whether or not they may be "adopted"—much like their developmentally-advanced counterparts—by infertile couples and given the chance to be born and raised in a loving family.

In *Dignitas Personae*, the Church has expressed serious reservations about embryo adoption, but did not explicitly condemn it. In view of this cautious attitude, Catholic theologians have been discussing the moral aspects of embryo adoption. Those who argue in favor of embryo adoption are careful to state that because a child already exists, it is a form of adoption, not a fertility treatment.[31] It does not restore reproductive health. They argue that it does not *assist* or *replace* intercourse; in fact, it has nothing to do with intercourse or reproduction at all. Theologians who argue against embryo adoption contend that it involves the future parents in an immoral process (IVF), it may lead to unfair discrimination among embryos (which to implant: only the healthy ones? only the male ones? only the Caucasian ones?), and would inevitably lead to the death of many embryos, since they would probably not all survive the thawing process. In the document *Dignitas Personae*, the Vatican made this statement:

> It has also been proposed, solely in order to allow human beings to be born who are otherwise condemned to destruction, that there could be a form of "*prenatal adoption*." This proposal, praiseworthy with regard to the intention of respecting and defending human life, presents however various problems. . . . All things considered, it needs to be recognized that the thousands of abandoned embryos represent a *situation of injustice which in fact cannot be resolved.* Therefore John Paul II made an "appeal to the conscience of the world's scientific authorities and in particular to doctors, that the production of human embryos be halted, taking into account that there seems to be no morally licit solution regarding the human destiny of the thousands and

thousands of 'frozen' embryos which are and remain the
subjects of essential rights and should therefore be protected by law as human persons."[32]

The moral problem involves the adoption of embryos that
were created in an immoral manner and potentially engages
many difficult moral, medical, psychological, and legal issues
for the genetic parents, for the child, and for the adoptive
parents. On the whole, it is a very complex issue that requires
thorough investigation before a decision can be made.

That is why the Church has very serious concerns about
the morality of embryo adoption. In reference to the document *Dignitas Personae,* the USCCB has said: "Proposals for
'adoption' of abandoned or unwanted frozen embryos are
also found to pose problems, because the Church opposes
use of the gametes or bodies of others who are outside the
marital covenant for reproduction. The document raises cau-
tions or problems about these new issues but does not
formally make a definitive judgment against them."[33] As a
result, Catholics who might consider it as a form of adoption
(not as a treatment for infertility) need to proceed with great
caution and with the expert counsel of a Catholic priest or
moral theologian qualified in this area.[34]

Hope in the Desert

Some of the medical alternatives discussed earlier that
are not morally acceptable (obtaining sperm through masturbation, heterologous procedures, ZIFT, ICSI, IVF, and
human cloning) may appear to treat infertility, but instead
they bypass the cause of our infertility and conceive a child
outside the union of husband and wife. Just as a mirage of
water offers false hope to a thirsty desert traveler, these

fertility treatments can offer false hope and pull us away from the course we should follow. Thirsty desert travelers often see mirages of water in the distance. Light rays bend in the extreme temperature differences that can often be found in different layers of desert air, and an image of the sky refracted onto the ground appears to be water. A person who is dying of thirst might consider doing anything to have a drink of that water, even if it is only a remote possibility. Likewise, we who have an unquenchable desire for a child and sometimes feel like we could die from longing often consider doing almost anything to conceive a child and maintain a healthy pregnancy. It is temptingly easy to allow our extreme emotions to bend the truth. When different medical alternatives dangle the possibility of a healthy pregnancy in front of us, even if it is only a remote possibility, we can find it extremely difficult to resist.

These morally unacceptable means are detours in the desert, paths that pull us away from God's will. Though they may often lead to pregnancy, they do so in a way that God does not intend. The ends do not justify the means. It is tempting to tell ourselves that God wants us to be happy, and that God desires that we should have children, and that maybe God would allow us to use ARTs since they may help us conceive. As we journey through the desert of infertility, we may constantly find ourselves coming back to the same question: What is God's will here? Our Catholic faith tells us that God never wills for us to do anything that is objectively morally wrong, and the ARTs listed above are objectively morally wrong. So, God's will must be something else.

The severe emotional suffering caused by infertility can lead to a mentality that says: "Pregnancy at all costs!" Indeed, the more time, money, and emotional energy we invest in trying to conceive and bear a healthy child—a very natural, good desire in and of itself—the more difficult it can be to make the decision to stop trying. We can begin to mistakenly believe that we have a right to a child, as if children are possessions. "The Church recognizes the legitimacy of the desire for a child and understands the suffering of couples struggling with problems of fertility. Such a desire, however, should not override the dignity of every human life to the point of absolute supremacy. The desire for a child cannot justify the 'production' of offspring . . ." through morally unacceptable means.[35] Children are gifts that cannot be demanded, but only received with awe and reverence from the hand of the true Artist of Life, God himself.

Yet, no matter how our children come to us, God is faithful. Whenever and however conception occurs, even if by an immoral means, God alone is the Creator and Redeemer of the human race. "For it is out of goodness—in order to indicate the path of life—that God gives human beings his commandments and the grace to observe them: it is likewise out of goodness—in order to help them persevere along the same path—that God always offers to everyone his forgiveness. Christ has compassion on our weaknesses: he is our Creator and Redeemer."[36]

Although certain reproductive technologies can never be morally acceptable, "every child who comes into the world must in any case be accepted as a living gift of the divine Goodness and must be brought up with love."[37] Children conceived through ART are not to blame for the circumstances surrounding their conception. Their parents love them, and the Church embraces them as children of God. Though their parents may have made an immoral decision, these children are gifts from God.

Many Catholic couples who have conceived children through ART did so without any prior knowledge of the Church's teachings. Under the extreme emotional distress that infertility brings, many Catholics make the best medical decisions they can based on the information they have at the time. "If a couple is unaware that the procedure is immoral, they are not subjectively guilty of sin."[38] However, they may still be troubled when they learn the Church's teachings concerning the way in which they chose to conceive their child. Further, there certainly are some Catholic couples who knew the Church's teachings before they conceived their children through ART, but never understood the rationale behind these teachings. This is why it is best for couples to be fully-informed about the Church's teachings on these matters and to understand the moral reasoning involved prior to pursuing treatment. While it is true that one must follow one's conscience, as Catholics we have the responsibility to form our consciences rightly according to the teachings of Christ and his Church. These teachings must not be taken lightly or dismissed because of an ardent desire to conceive a child.

While it is understandably difficult for parents to re-evaluate the decisions that brought them their children, moral integrity demands honesty. Though painful, it is possible and praiseworthy for a parent to look back on their choices—and not the children that resulted from those choices—and admit that they were wrong. Remorse for a decision to use ART does not imply that a parent regrets conception. On the contrary, it would be an act of selfless love for one's child to honestly evaluate the circumstances surrounding their conception and wish one had made better choices for them, choices that would have assigned to them the dignity they deserve.

If you find yourself in this situation, know that Jesus is waiting for you to turn to him in honesty and seek his healing love. Remember, *he loves you and longs for you even more than you long for a child.* He has been with you through your entire life. He knows your heart better than you do. Find a priest who is knowledgeable about these issues, and speak with him. If you were aware of the Church's teachings prior to conceiving your child, please prayerfully consider celebrating God's forgiveness in the sacrament of Confession. Nothing is outside the realm of God's forgiveness.

QUESTIONS FOR REFLECTION AND DISCUSSION

- Do you know how to recognize the naturally occurring signs of the fertile period in your (or your wife's) cycle? If not, you can receive training so you can use fertility-focused intercourse to try to achieve pregnancy. (See the resources in Appendix C.)

- What is your reaction upon learning that there is an entire medical institute dedicated to treating infertility that abides by the Church's moral teachings? Would you consider finding a NaProTECHNOLOGY doctor in your area or contacting the Pope Paul VI Institute for the Study of Human Reproduction for medical evaluation and treatment?

- Before reading this chapter, what was your understanding of the Church's teachings regarding ARTs? At that time, what did you think about these procedures? Now that you are fully aware of the Church's teachings regarding ARTs and the rationale behind these teachings, how do you evaluate these treatments?

ొ What would you like to share with your spouse from
    your reflection?

FOR FRIENDS AND FAMILY

It is incredibly difficult to watch a loved one suffer
through infertility. The medical decisions your loved one may
face are complicated and intricate, so naturally if you have
heard of something that you think might be helpful, your first
instinct may be to share that information. I would offer a
word of caution here. Just because a treatment was featured
on the news or it helped a friend of a friend does not mean it
would be appropriate for your loved one. However, solid
information is a good thing. Instead of offering your own
medical advice, it may be more helpful to just give them a
copy of this book. Then they can sort through the information on their own and be informed about all of their options
so they can work with their doctor (or find another doctor).

PRAYER

Teach me your way, O LORD,
    that I may walk in your truth;
    give me an undivided heart to revere your name.
I give thanks to you, O Lord my God, with my whole
        heart,
    and I will glorify your name forever.

Psalm 86:11–12

Chapter 5

Handling Anger

When Rachel saw that she bore Jacob no children, she envied her sister; and she said to Jacob, "Give me children, or I shall die!"

Genesis 30:1

When I went through infertility, I was very angry with God. I was thirty-eight when I met and fell in love with J. God had answered my prayers for a husband, just not on my timetable. My husband and I desperately wanted to have a child. Even though my mother and many other women in my family had given birth after the age of forty, I was not able to conceive. I felt like God was saying, "Nope. Not for you." It really hurt.

My anger clouded my perspective. I wanted to be pregnant and to have a baby, a child whose very being would reflect the love between me and my husband. If we couldn't have that, then I thought I could never be happy. That was my biggest problem with accepting infertility. But God showed me that I was wrong. He used my aunt, whose spirit was joyful despite years of tremendous personal suffering, to teach me that while I might always be sad about infertility, I could be happy in other ways. I gained some perspective, and we are very happy! God has given us the two children that he always intended to be ours through adoption, and we could not imagine our lives any other way. I am so grateful that God finally answered our prayers according to his plan, and not mine.

— B. J.

The Storm Clouds Gather

When harsh reality sets in and a couple acknowledges their infertility, perhaps choosing a doctor and initial course of treatment, anger usually dawns. When we can no longer deny our infertility, we may want to push it as far away from ourselves as we can. In the process, we can push away all those people and things that remind us of our pain. I avoided getting a haircut for almost a year because my hairdresser always asked me when I was going to have children. Finally I just found a new hairdresser. Sometimes people made thoughtless comments to my husband as well, remarks that were very hurtful. Unfortunately, it is impossible to escape pregnant strangers at the mall, babies at Mass, and Mother's Day and Father's Day—those dreaded days of mourning for couples struggling with infertility.

Another source of frustration and hurt often comes when couples reach out to family and friends for support. Instead, others may give the couple unwanted and useless advice. Suggestions can range from the ridiculous—"wear socks next time"—to the infuriating—"just relax, and it will happen." I'll never forget the day one doctor made this latter remark to me. I burst into tears as soon as she said it, and then I proceeded to tell her that I did not appreciate her advice and that I was not to blame for my infertility. An infertile friend of mine had a ready response for this situation. She would say, "Stress does not cause infertility; infertility causes stress." Relaxation disappears when intimacy with your spouse feels like it has turned into a science experiment.

The changes that happen to a couple's intimate life create added stress. Spouses may push each other away to elude the reality of their infertility. The worst arguments of a couple's marriage can happen at this point, and sadly, many good marriages may fall apart. The tension caused by infertility is like a huge, violent storm brewing in the desert, which can leave a path of emotional destruction in its wake. It can even be difficult to try to conceive during this phase of the journey because conception requires intercourse, and angry people don't make good company for one another. I can remember nights when I'd tell my husband, "I don't care if we're in the middle of a disagreement. I'm ovulating." Anger can be ridiculous at times.

Nonetheless, we often find it difficult to be angry with every fiber of our being and not to blame someone, somewhere. Many people begin to blame God for their infertility. After all, he is in charge, isn't he? And he's the one who blessed our first parents, Adam and Eve, saying: "Be fruitful and multiply." Many Catholics have been raised with the notion that God prefers big families. The *Catechism of the Catholic Church* states: "Sacred Scripture and the Church's traditional practice see in *large families* a sign of God's blessing and the parents' generosity."[1] The more children, it would seem, the better.

Couples often believe they are trying to do God's will by trying to conceive, but they feel frustrated when they encounter obstacle after obstacle. They can easily rationalize: "If God wanted me to be pregnant, I would be. Why is he punishing me?" While these thoughts and feelings are understandable, and while God can certainly handle the anger that may be directed toward him, it isn't God's fault. God does not desire or will infertility for anyone. God's control panel doesn't have a "thunderbolt" button. God desires only happiness for us, his beloved children.

Another complication often encountered at this juncture is that spouses react differently. One spouse may still be in denial, while the other has moved on to anger. Spouses may move back and forth between different feelings with the new wave of reality that each period brings, and find themselves handling their feelings in very dissimilar ways. While infertility affects the couple as a couple, it also affects the spouses individually. Each spouse had their own unique vision of what parenthood would be like, and so each suffers their own unique loss.

It can be very helpful at this point to seek a third party for emotional support, such as a priest or spiritual director who can provide a perspective that your spouse might not be able to give you. A spiritual director is like a prayer counselor who can help you understand your experience in light of your relationship with God and in the context of your faith. Perhaps your pastor or another member of you parish staff can recommend someone. If the first person you talk to isn't helpful, try someone else. Don't give up.

Prayer can also bring powerful healing. Begin to pray with your spouse, if you aren't already doing so. Ask your pastor to pray for you and to consider including prayers for infertile couples in the Universal Prayer at Mass from time to time, especially on Mother's Day and Father's Day, and during the Advent and Christmas seasons. If you haven't been to Confession in a while, consider celebrating this wonderful sacrament of healing. Even if you haven't been to Confession for many years, try not to be intimidated. Think of it as an opportunity to receive the loving embrace of your God, who longs for you with deep affection. Just tell the priest it's been a long time, and ask him for help. He'll tell you exactly what you need to do, and the feeling of healing that comes may surprise you.

Sharing your frustrations with an impartial listener can often bring about a slow diffusion of your anger as they bear your burden with you. However, you can and should keep the lines of communication open with your spouse and lean on one another. Often I found that when I was paralyzed by fear, my husband would be feeling hopeful. Or when he was angry, I had found a moment of peace. Sometimes one of us was able to give what the other needed. This give and take, this sharing of the burden, can bring you closer together, dispel some of your anger, and strengthen your marriage at the same time.

QUESTIONS FOR REFLECTION AND DISCUSSION

∾ Do you feel angry about infertility? If so, name all the aspects of it that you feel angry about.

∾ Describe exactly how you feel at the beginning, middle, and end of each cycle when you realize that you are not pregnant.

∾ What people and situations do you avoid because of infertility?

∾ Do you blame God for your infertility? Explain.

∾ Is there anyone in your parish whom you could talk to about your infertility? If not, how will you seek support?

∾ How has infertility affected your relationship with your spouse? If it is needed, are you willing to work together to bring about healing there? How can this be accomplished?

∾ What would you like to share with your spouse from your reflection?

FOR FRIENDS AND FAMILY

Though you may truly mean the best, please never say "Just relax, and it will happen." Nothing you say can help your loved one relax if they are stressed, and contrary to popular belief, no medical study has ever proven that stress causes infertility. This comment may seem like you are saying that it is their fault that they have not conceived, and of course you would never mean to imply that. And as for the last part, ". . . it will happen," well, that's a tough one. It might not happen. This is your loved one's deepest fear and the cause of the stress. It would be better to say, "If there is anything I can do, or if you ever want to talk, just let me know. I will be praying for you."

PRAYER

O LORD, God of my salvation,
    when, at night, I cry out in your presence,
let my prayer come before you;
    incline your ear to my cry.
For my soul is full of troubles,
    and my life draws near to Sheol.
I am counted among those who go down to the Pit;
    I am like those who have no help,
like those forsaken among the dead,
    like the slain that lie in the grave. . . .
O LORD, why do you cast me off?
    Why do you hide your face from me?
You have caused friend and neighbor to shun me;
    my companions are in darkness.

                                    Psalm 88:1–5a, 14, 18

Chapter 6

Coping with Sadness

Her husband Elkanah said to her, "Hannah, why do you weep? Why do you not eat? Why is your heart sad? Am I not more to you than ten sons?"

1 Samuel 1:8

After years of infertility, I conceived. When I found out I was pregnant, I was ecstatic with joy. But I miscarried my baby after six weeks of pregnancy. This event was so traumatic and devastating—all my joy at the bottom of a toilet bowl. I felt as though a tornado had ripped through my life, picked me up, and then hurled me back to earth without a parachute. I was sprawled across the pavement prying pieces of myself from its grip, trying to put myself back together. I was utterly alone in this struggle. I was exhausted and depressed.

I hated how weak I was. What would become of me if I failed to get up from the ground and recover, if darkness won my broken soul? My energy and motivation waxed and waned each month, as the hope of pregnancy turned into failure. Slowly, the bitterness of my futile efforts overshadowed my heart. I wanted to fight, but how? Who would be my strength, for I had very little. I prayed, "God help me. Please, please bless us with a baby again soon, and please let it live."

— M. L.

The Rains Finally Fall

Many couples struggling to conceive don't experience sadness right away. Fear, terror, doubt, uncertainty, shock, denial, anger—all these feelings leave little room for sadness in the beginning. But if we turn these feelings *over* to God instead of directing them *at* him, he will embrace us the moment we reach out to him for help. And in that embrace with God, we can finally allow our tears to fall like the rains of sadness in the desert. For months, my prayer life was reduced to five sobbing words: "Lord, I am so sad." I could pray no other prayer at all.

Sadness comes when couples stop pushing away the reality of their infertility and begin to acknowledge it. This sadness comes from the variety of losses involved with infertility, and each spouse may feel these losses to varying degrees. My deepest sadness was caused by the thought of missing the experience of pregnancy. I wanted to be pregnant so badly that I would dream about it at night, only to wake up to my sad reality. For some, the loss of continuing their family bloodline may cause the greatest sadness. For others, nothing could be worse than not being able to conceive a child with their spouse. The particular cause of sadness may differ for each spouse, but the feeling is the same.

Sadness may bring on physical symptoms as well: sleeplessness, or oversleeping; loss of appetite, or overeating; loss of interest in things that formerly brought happiness; lethargy and fatigue; physical aches and pains; nausea; and of course, prolonged bouts of crying. Spouses may begin staying up so late that they can just pass out from exhaustion, instead of facing the thoughts that may come to torture them after their head hits the pillow. Or they may never want to get out of bed. Some people lose or gain a significant amount of weight from poor eating habits. Others may stop socializing with friends or give up hobbies they used to love. It is very common to let things like cooking and laundry fall by the wayside. Some people begin to suffer tension headaches and neck or back pain. I felt sick all the time. Any minor argument with my husband sent waves of nausea over me. It was a cruel twist on morning sickness.

People suffering some of these severe symptoms may want to consider seeking professional help for depression. The medical community is beginning to recognize that many people going through infertility suffer from a form of clinical depression commonly referred to as infertility depression. In fact, women going through infertility have been shown to suffer depression at the same rates as women going through such life-threatening diseases as cancer and heart disease.[1] Seeking a professional counselor or therapist who specializes in treating patients suffering from infertility-induced depression may prove helpful for some people.

Some fertile friends and family members may not know what to say to us, and they may at times inadvertently hurt our feelings very deeply. These relationships may suffer for a while, but good friends will have compassion and want to know what they can do to help. It is understandable to decline invitations to baby showers and to steer clear of the maternity and baby sections of department stores, but some situations are hard to avoid. I burst into tears at Thanksgiving dinner when everyone innocently decided to watch a video of my baby nephew's first bath. I cried for nearly an hour. Most dreaded of all was that brief moment in the morning when my body was starting to wake up but my mind was a few steps behind, and for a few barely conscious moments I forgot that I was infertile, only to be hit by the cold sheet of ice water that was my new reality.

My oldest sister, a fellow traveler in this desert, once told me that infertility means learning how to live your life in the company of Sadness, which can become a quasi-being that takes on an existence all its own. This Sadness never completely leaves. Sometimes Sadness mercifully recedes to the shadowy corners of our life. At other times, and sometimes without warning, Sadness sits on our chest and steals our breath.

Sadness acknowledges the value of what is lost, and admits that it might be lost forever. I am sorry to report that very often, some aspects of sadness may never truly leave a couple unless they can achieve and sustain a healthy pregnancy. Just like the loss of a loved one can still make you sad decades after that person's death, so too can infertility. But this doesn't mean that you will spend every day weeping for the rest of your life. Even if you never conceive, the pain and sorrow will eventually dissipate to some extent. It takes a lot of time, and a lot of prayer. There's no way around it. You cannot avoid it. You simply have to walk straight through it.

It is in your heart's deep places of darkness, sadness, and emptiness that you can encounter Christ. Because he became fully human and loves you so much that he died for you, Christ completely understands the darkest reaches of your suffering. He already knows what you are going through, and he knows exactly how things are going to turn out. Whether or not you are interested in the grace Christ offers at any particular time, he will wait patiently for you to crawl into his embrace and sob.

I sobbed to Jesus for an hour every morning on my way to work, and for another hour on my way home. My spiritual director, very wise in the ways of women's hearts, asked me an interesting question. She wanted to know what aspect of Christ's life, what image of him from all the stories I'd ever heard at Mass or read in the Bible, did I feel the greatest connection to in my sadness. I felt drawn to the image of Christ in the desert. In my mind's eye, my husband and I were in the desert with Christ, and we were hopelessly lost. It was raining in the desert—a windy torrent of drenching water and driving sand. We had to close our eyes and bow our heads, bracing ourselves against the storm. In our grief, we couldn't see the path that lay ahead of us. All we could do was clumsily reach out to grasp one another with one hand, and desperately clutch at Christ's cloak with the other, stumbling after him into whatever the future held for us. Through prayer, Christ continually led me back to this image of following him through the desert. Though the path behind him was difficult, knowing that we were following our Lord gave us hope.

Questions for Reflection and Discussion

- ∞ Have you talked to your spouse about your feelings of sadness? Please elaborate.

- ∞ Since you began dealing with infertility, have any holidays passed that have been particularly difficult? Describe your experiences.

- ∞ Of all the losses associated with infertility described in chapter 1, which brings you the most sadness? Describe your feelings.

- ∞ From which, if any, of the physical symptoms of sadness do you suffer? How would you describe your spouse's sadness?

- ∞ What aspect of Christ's life—what image of him from all the stories you've ever heard at Mass or from your own reading of the Bible—do you feel the greatest connection to in your sadness? Describe this image, and let it remain with you in prayer.

- ∞ What would you like to share with your spouse from your reflection?

For Friends and Family

Be as sensitive as you can be to the sadness that your loved one may be experiencing. Events that are usually happy occasions for other people, such as holidays, baby showers, Mother's Day and Father's Day, birthdays, Baptisms, family parties—in short anything involving babies or young children—may be particularly difficult for them. Other people's happiness may sometimes remind them of their unhappiness. Please do not take offense if they decline invitations during the holidays or for events that involve children. Instead, try to spend time with them in some other way in which the focus is not on children.

Prayer

Be gracious to me, O Lord, for I am in distress;
  my eye wastes away from grief,
  my soul and body also.
For my life is spent with sorrow,
  and my years with sighing;
my strength fails because of my misery,
  and my bones waste away.
I am the scorn of all my adversaries,
  a horror to my neighbors,
an object of dread to my acquaintances;
  those who see me in the street flee from me. . . .
I have passed out of mind like one who is dead;
  I have become like a broken vessel.

Psalm 31:9–12

Chapter 7

Envy, Shame, Guilt, and Blame

After those days his wife Elizabeth conceived, and for five months she remained in seclusion. She said, "This is what the Lord has done for me when he looked favorably on me and took away the disgrace I have endured among my people."

LUKE 1:24–25

I couldn't understand why I had to go through infertility when it seemed like everyone around me was getting pregnant at the drop of a hat. Even though I wanted to be happy for my family members and friends when they conceived, I couldn't help but feel frustrated, resentful, and even angry at them because it seemed so unfair. I thought they were clueless when they would tell me their news without warning, when I had no place to hide my tearful reactions, or when they would complain to me about the aches and pains associated with pregnancy. I could only think, *How dare they? Don't they know how fortunate and blessed they are? What I wouldn't give to experience morning sickness or swollen ankles!*

I wracked my brain trying to think of all the things I could blame myself for, things that would account for my infertility. I felt so guilty for being less of a woman for my husband and for being unable to build a family together. And I felt incredibly selfish for not wanting to adopt. Even though so many wonderful children in the world need good parents, all I craved was the experience of being pregnant with a child that my husband and I had conceived together.

I kept asking God, "Why me?" Why did it feel like God was ignoring my prayers and abandoning me? Wasn't God the one being I felt I could always turn to and depend on? Hadn't I been a good Catholic and lived a moral life? Hadn't I always hung onto my faith, no matter how often it had been tested in the past? Why couldn't God just give us a baby? I felt like God was punishing me for something I must have done. During a particularly emotional commute to work one morning, when all of these questions were swirling in my head, I felt an amazing sense of calm fall over me. It finally dawned on me that no matter how much I thought I was in control of this process, it was not up to me. It was all in God's hands. It was in his plan whether or not I would become a mother some day.

Even though that idea was still very hard for me to accept, it allowed me to relax a little. It also allowed me to forgive myself for all the feelings of envy, shame, guilt, and blame I was having. I realized that it was okay and only natural to feel that way. I also became more empathetic toward other women going through infertility. I am now a team member for a great fertility support group in my church. But most of all, having experienced these feelings allowed me to fully enjoy every moment of my pregnancy and the birth and life of my daughter. When I look at her every day, I know why it was best to wait for God's time. And I can't imagine it any other way.

— M. G.

Beholding Our Own Brokenness

The image of Christ in the desert gradually became a source of comfort for me. Even if I didn't know where I was going, Christ did. Yet, I also felt drawn to Christ as I imagined him robed and crowned with thorns—the image of him being mocked and shamed by his torturers on his way to the cross. At first, this image surprised me. Then I realized that I felt mocked and shamed by my own body.

Shame and embarrassment often come with infertility. They are normal parts of sadness. It is typical for one or both spouses to feel ashamed. The wife feels ashamed because she cannot become pregnant, or the husband feels ashamed because he cannot father his wife's child. Both may feel that their bodies have failed at the most significant task it is designed to accomplish. A man may feel as if he is somehow less of a man, while a woman may feel she is less of a woman. Of course, this isn't true. Yet, the powerful feelings of shame, guilt, inadequacy, embarrassment, incompetence, and even defectiveness remain, and these feelings can have a powerful impact on a couples' intimacy. These feelings can be heightened if infertility comes after a sexually transmitted disease, a previous abortion,[1] or past use of contraceptives.

Though these factors are certainly not always present, they can contribute to infertility. Diseases that are still not openly discussed, such as chlamydia and gonorrhea, often lead to infertility.[2] Unfortunately, the stigma attached to these and other STDs is perhaps even greater than the stigma attached to infertility. Perhaps it is a small favor that these diseases are notoriously hard to trace, especially if both spouses are infected and have a history of sexual activity outside of marriage. Additionally, though most women who suffer the loss of a child through abortion are never told this, abortion may affect future fertility.[3] It can be emotionally devastating for a woman to look back on a past pregnancy that she chose to terminate, and realize it may have led to her present infertility. Finally, although not common, past use of oral contraceptives can also contribute to infertility.[4]

At this point it is easy to fall into either blaming yourself or blaming your spouse, but that is a temptation to avoid. Sometimes a particular diagnosis makes it tempting to blame either one person or the other. One might blame oneself, thinking, *If I hadn't insisted on waiting so long to start trying, maybe we would have been able to conceive. It's my fault.* Or worse, one might harbor resentment against one's spouse, thinking, *If she hadn't had sex with so many people before we got married, maybe she wouldn't have contracted the infection that made her infertile. It's her fault.* Many men and women who lost a child through a previous abortion find it very difficult to see their way out of the darkness of their feelings of regret and guilt.[5]

While all of these feelings are normal and understandable, they accomplish nothing good and have the potential to be very harmful. Blaming yourself can destroy your own sense of self-worth and lead to serious depression, and blaming your spouse can destroy your marriage. Yet, as painful as it may be, you and your spouse need to honestly communicate to preserve your marriage from being undermined by guilt, blame, and resentment. If you discover the medical reason for your infertility and realize how your past actions may have brought it about, it is helpful to honestly acknowledge whatever responsibility you may bear for it. I am not suggesting that you demand an accounting from your spouse. But if it becomes apparent that one or both of you have something to admit, let it see the light of day and be healed by the light of Christ. Turn to God's loving mercy in the sacrament of Reconciliation, confess your fault, and find forgiveness. Forgive yourself and/or forgive your spouse, and let go of the guilt and blame. Do not allow resentful thoughts to rent space in your head or heart any longer. Instead, think of infertility as a medical difficulty that you endure together.

Even if past use of contraception, an STD, or a past abortion are not to blame, it is in this moment of utter brokenness and devastation, when we realize our own personal inadequacies, that Christ desires to embrace us with his healing and unconditional love. The sacraments of Confession and perhaps Anointing of the Sick may be particularly helpful at this time. We may think that this last sacrament is reserved exclusively for those who are dying. This is not the case. Anyone whose health is seriously impaired by sickness or who is about to undergo surgery may celebrate this sacrament. Let your priest decide if you may receive this sacrament, or if he can celebrate the Order for the Blessing of the Sick. All of these rituals allow us to reach out to Christ and ask for whatever kind of healing we think we need. Be assured, if you are open to whatever grace Christ has to offer, he will heal you in the way you most need, even if this isn't the way you most desire.

QUESTIONS FOR REFLECTION AND DISCUSSION

- Envy and resentment are not the most socially acceptable feelings, yet it is normal for us to experience them when we are going through infertility. Describe any situations in which you have felt envious or resentful of another's happiness.

- What role, if any, does shame or guilt play in your experience of infertility?

- Do you blame yourself for your infertility? Do you blame your spouse? Do you have any valid reason to assign such blame? Do you have reason to believe that your infertility may have resulted from anything that you or your spouse have done in the past? How can you honestly discuss this with your spouse in a way that brings about healing and not harm?

- When was the last time you went to Confession? How do you feel about this sacrament now? Would you consider trying it?

- How do you feel about the sacrament of Anointing of the Sick? If you are hesitant, you can ask your pastor about it.

- What would you like to share with your spouse from your reflection?

For Friends and Family

Many people wonder if and how to share the most wonderful news of their lives—that they are pregnant—with a friend or family member struggling with infertility. Though the news may or may not be privately painful for them to hear, they should be among the first people you tell. You would not want them to hear it from someone else and be caught off guard, wondering why you didn't tell them yourself. If you hope to make a big announcement at a large gathering, you may want to let your loved one know first. It may be important to tell them privately if you think they might be self-conscious about how their reaction is perceived by others. Be as sensitive as you can be, and try not to have any expectations. They may not be able to give you an overjoyed reaction, or they may surprise you.

Prayer

In you, O Lord, I seek refuge;
  do not let me ever be put to shame;
  in your righteousness deliver me.
Incline your ear to me;
  rescue me speedily.

Psalm 31:1–2a

Chapter 8

Setting Limits and Reaching Acceptance

Now there was a woman who had been suffering from hemorrhages for twelve years. She had endured much under many physicians, and had spent all that she had; and she was no better, but rather grew worse. She had heard about Jesus, and came up behind him in the crowd and touched his cloak, for she said, "If I but touch his clothes, I will be made well."

MARK 5:25–28

My husband and I struggled with unexplained infertility for three years. It started with ovulation predictor sticks and temperature charts, but before I knew it we were doing injections and daily ultrasounds, which were followed by failed treatment cycles. My reproductive endocrinologist finally told my husband and me that without *in vitro* fertilization we had less than a 4 percent chance of conceiving on our own.[1]

Our insurance didn't cover the extremely high cost of each IVF cycle, and each attempt offered only a 20 percent chance of success. We couldn't afford to gamble. Instead, we decided to increase our chances with more aggressive medication. I knew that I was risking a pregnancy with multiples, but all I cared about was getting pregnant. Instead of conceiving, I developed multiple ovarian cysts from all the injections. That's when I completely lost it. I broke down and cursed my doctor and everyone else in the room. Thank goodness my doctor was very compassionate and wasn't the least bit offended.

I will never forget the ride home from the doctor's office that day. My husband turned to me and said, "That's it. We're done with this." I thank God that he was able to see the end, because I might not have given up. And who knows what that would have done to our marriage and my mental health. We went home and took some time to grieve the loss of the biological child we would never have. Soon we put in our application to adopt from Korea. Sixteen months later my beautiful son flew halfway around the world and into my arms forever.

Ironically, less than a year later I gave birth to my first biological son. I went on to have two more biological children without any infertility treatments. So I have beaten my less than 4 percent odds three times now. I like to think that my infertility led me to the path of adoption, which ultimately led me to my first son. I cannot imagine my life without him.

— J. A.

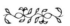

Searching for Limits—
Where Does the Desert End?

Many couples find it helpful to take temporary breaks or to set some kind of a limit on how long they are willing to try to conceive, how much money they are willing to spend, or how much emotional suffering they are willing to endure. Many people also limit what kinds of treatments they are willing to consider. Many times these self-imposed limits are the only reason couples are able to move on with their lives.

Though it may seem strange to say this, my husband and I were fortunate to have been told quite clearly that we would never conceive a child. The reproductive issues that both of us had were enough for our doctor to eliminate biological parenthood as a possibility without doing IVF. We had already excluded this and certain other fertility treatments from what we were willing to do, so when we were told that only those options would work, we knew that pregnancy had been taken off the table. We were told that no other treatments were available, and that even if we had therapeutic surgeries, we would still not conceive. We had no drug to take, no procedure to try, no magical incantation to utter. *Nothing* would work.

Looking back, I now realize that it was a blessing to be spared the agony that many people go through of having to stop pursuing pregnancy after years of failed attempts. Our diagnosis saved us from the anguish of looking back and thinking, *What if we had tried for another year?* We had nothing to try. There simply was no way we would ever conceive a child. (This is what our doctors told us, anyway. God had other ideas when he created our second son.)

I was also blessed to have experienced adoption firsthand, having an older brother and sister whom my parents adopted before my other sister and I were born. Building a family through adoption was not the huge leap for me that it is for many people. My husband and I had actually talked about it when we were engaged, and we had toyed with the idea of pursuing adoption after we had a few biological children. Years later, when we thought we would never have biological children, we moved on to what might have been the next phase of our family plan anyway.

However, many couples experiencing prolonged infertility and/or repeated miscarriage have the daunting task of setting limits on their pursuit of pregnancy. Of course, many people don't set any limits in the beginning, because limits imply that the treatments may not work. Many people will not even consider the possibility of permanent infertility—their worst fear—until they have reached their personal emotional threshold for pain. As each failed cycle plummets couples deeper and deeper into the pit of human suffering and grief, each new attempt pulls them farther up into the realm of fragile hope. The deeper into sadness you fall, the higher your spirit must be lifted in order to entertain hope.

Each month that passes without conception brings ever-greater despair, more and more delicate hope, and an ever-growing, unquenchable desire for a child. The longer a couple cannot conceive, the deeper their sadness grows, and the more fragile their hope becomes. Yet after one treatment has been exhausted, another may be waiting. Hope springs eternal once again, and the emotional roller coaster takes off for a second spin, or a third, or a fourth. This struggle may be compounded by a change in health coverage or a couple's financial situation.

Another situation arises when couples struggling through infertility experience the additional and quite different loss of miscarriage. When a couple does finally succeed in conceiving a child, their hope soars. They may excitedly tell people that they are *finally* pregnant! Their lives are changed forever. They can finally begin to let go of the pain of infertility and experience unadulterated joy for the first time since their journey began. They have come to the end and feel like human beings again. A new day has dawned when at last they can find the happiness of being parents. They can finally begin to plan for the future and rekindle old hopes that had seemed so far away.

It is impossible to imagine the agony these couples endure when a miscarriage snatches the life of their child. Anyone who has not suffered firsthand through this pain can never truly understand it.

If the couple decides to continue trying to conceive, the emotional roller coaster ride can start all over again and may even grow worse. Now they may believe they have a greater reason to keep trying, since it worked before. And now that they have experienced a pregnancy, they may desire it even more than ever. Their future was within reach, yet slipped away. They also may approach each attempt differently. Like all who experience infertility, they are terrified that it won't work and hopeful that it will. But now they are also terrified that even if they do conceive, they may again experience the pain of miscarriage. So even if they are able to conceive, they may struggle to build hope and find it difficult to experience unadulterated happiness about their pregnancy until they have a healthy newborn baby in their arms.

Whether or not you have experienced miscarriage, and whether or not you already have a child or children prior to experiencing secondary infertility, your current attempts to conceive a child will eventually come to an end. Either you will conceive and have a healthy pregnancy, or you will not. These are the only two possible outcomes. Unfortunately, the only way to truly know if you could possibly ever get pregnant in this life is to have at your disposal unlimited financial, emotional, and medical resources and continue trying until you reach menopause. Even if you don't want to impose any limits on your attempts to conceive, your body will. And the reality is that most couples' financial and emotional resources—let alone their marriage—wouldn't last nearly half that long.

Those who do not conceive and give birth to a healthy baby in the short term have to consider what their limits are. Something has to give at some point, which will be different for every couple. Some couples realize early on that their financial situation will impose its own limit. But this isn't the only consideration. Many couples are unwilling to try certain medical treatments, due to either their religious commitments or their own personal discomfort with the treatments. Other couples may become aware of their own emotional limitations as time goes on and decide that in order to preserve their marriage and their emotional well-being, they have to set an endpoint. For many couples, age may become a factor, not only for medical reasons, but because many adoption programs have age restrictions. For some couples, adoption and foster parenting are simply not options—for whatever reason—and a decision to stop trying to conceive means that they will never become parents.

Once you have a solid diagnosis and your treatment options are put before you, it would be unwise to keep trying to conceive with no end in sight. Any worthy doctor would not recommend that you do so. Instead, couples may want to sit down and have an open, caring, and sensitive discussion about how to plan an endpoint if things should come to that. Your decision depends on your diagnosis, your financial situation, your emotional and spiritual stamina, your ability to put your life on hold in many ways, and, most importantly, the state of your marriage. Is it getting stronger or weaker? Your marriage must always come first—it is more important than getting pregnant in any given cycle. If one of you needs to take a break for a cycle, talk about it. If one of you is reaching the end before the other, talk about it. Though the process may be difficult and rife with arguments, though it may require an infertility counselor or therapist, and though it takes much prayer begging God to make his will clear, most couples finally come to a mutual understanding about when to stop trying to conceive.

Hopefully you will conceive and have a healthy pregnancy before that endpoint comes. If you do not, however, it is important to set a mutually agreed upon limit and stick to it. Decide in advance if it is the end of the road, or just a pit stop. People sometimes need to take breaks in order to continue trying to conceive. Other couples would never dream of taking a break and continue trying with all their might.

Unfortunately, since we cannot forecast the future, we will never know how things would have turned out if we had made a different decision. And that can be hard to accept. But we can be comforted, even if only a little, in knowing that we are making a decision that will disentangle ourselves from the monthly roller-coaster ride of infertility treatment and allow us to walk into our future, whatever it may hold.

Once we reach the limits of what we are willing to endure to conceive a child and decide to stop trying, we can finally begin to grieve our infertility completely. The experience is similar to that of a family that has a member with a terminal illness. This loved one may have gone through many cycles of illness and recovery, bringing hope and despair with each turn of health. When this loved one finally dies, the family feels great grief and loss, but they experience a certain amount of relief as well. They can now let go of their loved one and move into the future without that person, having come to terms with their loss.

In the same way, couples who decide to stop trying to conceive can finally grieve the loss of never having a biological child (or another one). They can say good-bye once and for all to that particular future and know that they will never again have to do so. Though this pain and sorrow may cause them deep grief, at least the wound it leaves is not reopened every month. It can finally begin to heal. Yes, it will leave a scar, and, like all scars, it may hurt more at some times than at others, but it will never again be torn open.

If you come to the end of your battle with infertility without the gift of a child, it is important to give yourself tremendous credit for your efforts in the struggle. You are a survivor. Infertility is not a terminal condition. Though at times it feels as if it may, infertility cannot kill you. And at the risk of seeming trite, what doesn't kill you makes you stronger. Take it from one who saw the endpoint come and go. No one but you, your spouse, and Jesus knows the particular road that you have been on.

Acceptance

Now is the time to take stock of your journey and remember it in the presence of Christ. The end of infertility treatment is the beginning of finally accepting the loss of biological children. You may wish to go back to Chapter 1 to review the most painful aspects of your loss, and then give them to Christ. Allow yourself the freedom to wish with all your heart that things would have turned out differently, but do the grief work necessary to accept your loss. Do not set any boundaries on your journey toward healing, and accept the fact that your cross of infertility may feel light at times, but at other times it may feel like it will crush you. Christ accepted his cross—indeed, he willingly embraced it with great love for all humanity—but I think we can safely assume that he wasn't excited about it. He didn't look forward to the physical pain of his death. He didn't walk cheerfully down the road to Golgotha. He walked slowly—barely able to stand under the weight of his suffering. The Stations of the Cross, a Catholic devotion focusing on Christ's suffering and death, tell us that Christ fell three times on the way to his execution and needed another man, Simon of Cyrene, to help him carry his cross.

Our loving Lord doesn't expect any more from us in carrying our burden of infertility. Acceptance simply means that, with God's grace, we take up our cross and follow Christ wherever he leads us. Remember that Jesus will never let you carry your cross alone.[2] He has been on this journey with you, guiding you through the desert since you entered it. You have lived through this experience with him and have the scars to prove it.

Oddly enough, the physical scars left on my abdomen from my surgeries make the shape of a cross. Every time I see them they remind me that I have been crucified with Christ. If you can accept your cross of infertility and unite your suffering to his, you will be crucified with him as well. And we know that ". . . if we have died with Christ, we believe that we will also live with him" (Rom 6:8). Those who die with Christ

rise to new life with Christ. Jesus can take the broken pieces
of your heart and create a new heart. He can give you a new
future, a future better than the one you had imagined for
yourself. But he can only do it if you remain connected to
him and desire new life with him. When we accept our cross
of infertility and finally say good-bye to the future we hoped
would be ours, we make ourselves available to another
future—the future God will lead us into after this time of trial
and suffering.

My oldest sister Martha's experience of infertility may
shed some light here. She successfully conceived and bore a
healthy son after at least two years of struggling through
infertility. Almost every month for the next ten years she
struggled again to conceive another child. I can't even remember the number of surgeries and treatments she had. She
conceived twice during that time, and miscarried twice.

Her experience of grief and loss began taking its toll, and
she finally allowed herself the freedom to move on. Her final
treatment cycle came before a significant birthday, and so she
decided to make that year the first year of the rest of her life.
She had a very special party for herself. She invited all of her
closest girlfriends, sent beautiful invitations, and hired a
wonderful catering company. Before the party she said to me,
"I will have one of two announcements to make at this party.
Either this last attempt will have succeeded and I'll tell everyone that I'm pregnant; or this last attempt will have failed and
I will tell everyone that I'm done. Either way, I am so excited,
because I feel like whatever happens will finally be God's will.
And even if it's hard, that's what I really want."

Deciding to be done with infertility doesn't mean it's done
with you, however. Even after we stop trying to conceive, and
we allow ourselves to grieve our loss deeply and completely,

the pain of infertility can still come up. It leaves a scar on our hearts that can smart at times. Even after my husband and I had proceeded with our adoption plans, I found myself sobbing on my bedroom floor after I talked to my sister Mary as she rode to the hospital in labor with my nephew. I was still excited about adopting, but I suddenly realized that I would never have that exciting experience of rushing to the hospital in labor (at the time I didn't realize how exciting rushing to the airport to pick up my son would be). For a long time I couldn't walk past the maternity section in a department store without getting upset. I considered it a victory to be able to go to a baby shower without breaking into tears.

Though I did conceive quite unexpectedly, I was on strict bedrest for three months in constant pre-term labor, rushing to the hospital near miscarriage on an almost weekly basis. My second son is lucky to be alive, and I have no reason to believe that his conception wasn't a completely unrepeatable coincidence. We adopted our third child not only because we loved the experience of adopting and couldn't wait to do it again, but also because we were not ready to go back through the possibility of infertility, another near-miscarriage, more bedrest, or worse—an actual miscarriage. Our daughter is now three years old, and we've been trying to conceive a fourth child for over a year. We've started treatment with a NaProTECHNOLOGY doctor, and are cautiously hopeful. Infertility the second time around is just as horrible as it was the first time. I know if I do conceive, I will worry about complications. Infertility still isn't done with me. It is still a cross I carry.

When I announced at my parish that I was beginning a new ministry with couples struggling through infertility, some couples in their sixties and seventies came up to me after Mass. With tears in their eyes, they told me that they wished there had been such a ministry for them when they were going through infertility. And these were people who later went on to have children, either biologically or through adoption. I had touched the scars infertility had left them with, and they felt sad all over again. But everyone is different. One of my girlfriends who had to have a complete hysterectomy and adopted her two boys has told me that she doesn't care in the least that she can't get pregnant. I am connected to many others whose lives have been touched by infertility and know that many people feel the way she does. That hasn't been my experience, but if you decide to stop trying to conceive, it may be yours.

When you decide to stop trying to conceive, you have to face another major decision. Do you and your spouse still want to be parents or not? More appropriately, do you believe that God is calling you to parenthood, or do you think God may be calling you to life as a family of two? If biological parenthood is no longer an option, God is definitely calling you to one of these alternatives. They are the only remaining choices. Both are wonderful opportunities to live a life full of love and possibility. You can find happiness in either of these options. If we have learned anything in the desert, however, we have learned that true happiness only comes from trusting in God. We can rely on him to lead us into the future he desires for us. In order to do this, we must not rush into anything. Instead, we can allow ourselves the opportunity to come to terms with the loss of biological children and prayerfully discern our future. If we quiet ourselves we will be able to hear his voice. This might be a wonderful time to take a relaxing vacation with your spouse or to go on a retreat. As you weigh your options and pray about your future, God will lead you to the path he wants you to take.

Questions for Reflection and Discussion

- ﹏ Right now, can you imagine yourself setting limits on what you are willing to do to conceive a child?
- ﹏ What financial limits do you face as you try to conceive? Are there any medical procedures that you are unwilling to undergo? How much longer can you imagine yourself trying to conceive?
- ﹏ Describe in detail the scenario in which you would be willing to consider setting an endpoint on your pursuit of pregnancy. What might that endpoint look like?
- ﹏ What do you think would be the most painful part of ending your pursuit of pregnancy, both for you and for your spouse?
- ﹏ Can you imagine yourself feeling relieved to walk away from your battle with infertility without the gift of a biological child? What about your spouse?
- ﹏ What would you like to share with your spouse from your reflection?

For Friends and Family

Couples struggling with infertility are forced to make difficult choices about what they are able and willing to endure to conceive. Morality, biology, emotions, marital strength, and finances all factor into a couples' decision to limit or end treatment for infertility. The most helpful thing friends and family can do is to remain positive and supportive of your loved ones, whether or not you agree with their decisions or would make the same choices for yourself. It really is a very personal and subjective experience. If you find that their decisions in this regard are eliciting a powerful emotional response in you, try not to allow your feelings to add to their already heavy burden.

PRAYER

Hear my prayer, O LORD;
  give ear to my supplications in your faithfulness;
  answer me in your righteousness. . . .
my spirit faints within me;
  my heart within me is appalled. . . .
I stretch out my hands to you;
  my soul thirsts for you like a parched land.
Answer me quickly, O LORD;
  my spirit fails.
Do not hide your face from me,
  or I shall be like those who go down to the Pit.
Let me hear of your steadfast love in the morning,
  for in you I put my trust.
Teach me the way I should go,
  for to you I lift up my soul.

Psalm 143:1, 4, 6–8

Chapter 9

Considering Adoption
and Other Options

"Whoever welcomes one such child in my name welcomes me."

MATTHEW 18:5

After three years of intensive fertility treatment, my husband and I decided to call it quits. The process caused too much stress and disappointment. Every month was like a funeral. We decided that adoption was our best route to parenthood. It was a bitter-sweet decision—bitter because we would never look into the face of a child who had my husband's eyes or my smile, and sweet because we could finally have our own child who was conceived in our hearts.

The adoption process was fairly easy. After only seven months we finished the interviews with the caseworker and doctor, and the home study was completed. Then the phone rang. "Hello, this is your adoption agency. We have a little six-week old boy who seems to be a good match for you. Would you like to pick him up?" I slid to the floor and croaked out the word, "When?" I was told, "Tomorrow at 9 A.M." I said, "Yes!" Then I made phone calls and ran to stores and friends to purchase or borrow what we needed for our son.

When I saw him for the first time, he seemed like a little bird that fell out of his nest. He was so tiny! My feelings were different from what I had expected. I felt like the baby sitter, not the mom. I kept looking over my shoulder whenever we left the house. I was so afraid that his birth mother would change her mind and want him back. But a few weeks later that all changed. I walked into his room to get him up and he looked at me and smiled and cooed while his little hands and feet were flying. He was happy to see me! At that moment I became "Mom" and no power on this earth could have separated us.

Five summers later we repeated the process. This time a five-month-old baby girl was waiting to meet us. Our experience with her was quite different. She was so big that she didn't fit into any of the clothes I had bought for her. She was so feisty that she tried to take my ice cream cone away from me on the ride home!

I felt completely fulfilled—well, almost. I could not have been more satisfied with my children or my life, but I still had one pang. The most natural experience for a woman is to be pregnant and give birth. What was wrong with me? I prayed and prayed that it would happen. Then one day I said, "God, I'm not praying for this anymore. You know better than I what I need. So, it's up to you." The next month, after sixteen years of unexplained infertility, I became pregnant with our third child. Then two years later we delivered our fourth.

One person very close to me asked me after my first biological child was born, "Well how does it feel to be a real mother?" I felt like she had put a knife in my heart. The love I had for all my children—adopted or biological—was the same even though I would whisper in all their ears when they were very little that they were each my favorite. I would forget from time to time that my first two were adopted. One day the pediatrician, while examining my oldest child, asked if anyone in the family had allergies. I mentioned that my mother and my uncle did. I didn't realize until I got home and talked to my mother that it was irrelevant. She had forgotten too. Your children are your children, no matter how God brings them to you, and a mother's love knows no bounds.

— G. D.

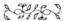

Discerning Adoption

After deciding to stop pursuing biological parenthood, adoptive parenthood and foster parenthood are the only roads left to having children. Many well-meaning but misguided people often tell those who are struggling with infertility to "just adopt," as if deciding to adopt a child instead of pursuing pregnancy is as easy as deciding to eat oatmeal for breakfast when you run out of cornflakes. For many people in the midst of infertility, even considering adoption feels like they have somehow betrayed their dedication to their long-hoped-for biological child. After investing so much time, energy, and resources into trying to conceive, considering adoption opens a door into an entirely new and unfamiliar future.

Before we consider adoption as a possible route to parenthood, we can look to our faith for guidance. Adoption is at least as old as civilization and has a long and very positive history in our faith tradition. When the Israelites were enslaved in Egypt and the Pharaoh ordered that all male children born to them should be killed, a Hebrew slave woman conceived and bore a son. She hid him for three months and then placed him in a waterproof basket among the reeds on the bank of the Nile River. The Pharaoh's daughter found him, adopted him as her son, and named him Moses (see Ex 2).[1] He would later lead the Israelites out of slavery. God chose Moses as his servant, the one through whom God established his covenant with the Israelites on Mount Sinai. Later in the Old Testament we hear of Queen Esther, who had been adopted by her cousin after her parents died (see Esther 2:7). God used Esther to bring deliverance to the Jewish people.

In the New Testament we learn of a young woman who found herself with child through the power of the Holy Spirit. Her betrothed husband, though he was not the child's biological father, brought her into his home and fostered the child, raising him as his own. Saint Joseph was the only human father Jesus ever had, and was no less his father even though he did not conceive him with the Blessed Mother (see Lk 1:35). Saint Joseph cheered the first steps Jesus took, heard his first babbling words, and taught him how to be a good Jewish man. He trained his foster son, our Lord, in his trade of carpentry, and, along with the Blessed Mother, raised him as his own son.

The Bible also uses adoption language to describe our relationship with God. In Romans 8:14–17 we read: "For all who are led by the Spirit of God are children of God. For you did not receive a spirit of slavery to fall back into fear, but you have received a spirit of adoption. When we cry, 'Abba Father!' it is that very Spirit bearing witness with our spirit that we are children of God, and if children, then heirs, heirs of God and joint heirs with Christ—if, in fact, we suffer with him so that we may also be glorified with him." There is no doubt that we are really God's children through adoption. In the sacrament of Baptism, God adopts each of us as his own child, and we become brothers and sisters of Jesus.

Even though adopting children is pleasing to God, and the Catholic Church recommends it, adoption is not for everyone. Adoption is a distinct call from God and should be discerned prayerfully as such. Though I don't feel this way myself, many people cannot wrap their minds and hearts around loving and raising a child whom they did not conceive. They simply cannot imagine themselves ever embracing this idea, and it is not wrong to feel this way. It would be best for such persons not to adopt, even if they wish they felt otherwise.

However, many other people are cautiously open to adoption but have doubts and questions. For most people, adopting a child requires a certain leap out of one's comfort zone, at least initially. Many people who come to adoption after experiencing infertility would admit that they would never have considered adoption if they had been able to conceive. Though they certainly wouldn't say it was a second-best choice, they would probably acknowledge it wasn't their first choice. Yet, having their child in their arms, they say this with gratitude to God for the cross of infertility. For if they had been able to conceive, they would not have become the parents to this beautiful child who is now their child, their love, their sweet angel without whom they cannot imagine their lives.

When couples first start to think about adoption, it often happens that one spouse becomes more comfortable with the idea before the other one does. This usually has to do with their differing experiences of infertility, which may affect their attitude toward adoption. For example, genetic continuity or family bloodlines may mean more to one spouse than the other. Spouses whose diagnosis was the primary cause of infertility may feel as if they have no right to stand in the way of their spouse becoming a parent through adoption, and they may fail to examine their own feelings adequately and honestly.

It is crucial for both spouses to communicate openly and honestly with one another about adoption, and this often requires taking a good look together at what infertility losses hurt the most. It may be helpful at this point to go back to the questions after Chapter 1 and discuss them with your spouse. Adoption does not cure infertility; it cures childlessness. This reality has to be owned by both spouses in order to be fair to any future children that come into your family through adoption. An adopted child is not a replacement for a biological child. Even if a child you adopt happens to look like you or can pass as your biological child, that child is a unique person in his or her own right. You know this, the child does or will know this, and anyone with whom you share this information will know this. That child is a genetically separate and unique human being with his or her own biological parents, cultural background, and medical history, and you cannot pretend otherwise. However, once you adopt, that child really is your child—your own child. You are his or her real mother and father.

While adoption does not give you the ability to conceive a child with your spouse, it does give both of you the ability to bring a child into your family. While one spouse often bears most of the paperwork load, it really is a shared experience. Many people call it a "paper pregnancy." It is a different journey than pregnancy, but it is a journey that you take together. And toward the end, before the child comes home, you will be swept into a crazy, chaotic rush of anxiety and last minute details that truly is its own labor.

So how is adoption different from biological parenthood, and how is it the same? Many people who have adopted children will tell you that kids are kids, no matter how they come to you. They will say that being a parent to a child who comes to you through adoption is no different than being a parent to a child who comes to you through conception. I have two children through adoption and one child through pregnancy, and I can tell you that there are mostly no differences after your children come home. Almost everything important is the same about raising them and being their parents. The only difference is that children who come into families through adoption bring with them the loss of their biological roots, and perhaps the loss of the culture or country into which they were born. Adoption is a life-long process and, as your adopted children grow and mature, their adoption story will weave an additional thread into the fabric of who they are and who you are as a family.

You certainly love your children through adoption just as much as you would biological children, no less and no more. Sometimes people who adopt try to argue that they are less likely to take their children for granted than those who conceive their children, but I don't think this is fair. We can't make such judgments about others, as if two different kinds of parents exist—biological and adoptive—and one is more loving than the other. Unfortunately, it's just as easy for us adoptive parents to lose patience, have less than stellar moments, and make mistakes.

Some aspects of the adoption process can feel much different from preparing for biological parenthood, especially in the time before your children are home. One thing that's different about adoption versus pregnancy is that you get to have your body back. During infertility treatment many women experience weight changes, and many medicines prescribed to treat infertility have unpleasant physical side effects. It was nice to lose all the weight that I had gained from going through infertility (and then some) and slip into a previously unimaginable size. I could work out as much and as hard as I wanted to. My sex life with my husband regained its meaning as an opportunity for us to renew our marriage bond and ceased feeling like a science experiment. After we decided to adopt, a small, very vain and shallow part of me relished the idea of looking incredible at my son's Baptism, when most women would still be larger than usual from pregnancy. Pretty ridiculous, I know, but I was reaching at that point. You can be an expectant parent and—within reasonable limits—drink alcohol, caffeine, and eat sushi when you adopt. You'll have no morning sickness and no swollen ankles.

But there's no swollen belly, no cute maternity clothes, and no strangers congratulating you on your expectancy. No one knows you are an expectant parent when you decide to adopt. You don't get to announce "I'm expecting!" in exactly the same way, because the adoption process is so different from pregnancy, and people often don't know what to say when you tell them. Should they feel bad for you because they know you had really wanted to be pregnant, or should they be happy for you because you are finally going to become a parent?

I remember being underwhelmed when I announced my good news to one of my girlfriends. She didn't know how to react and made a remark that would have been more appropriate if I had told her we had decided to get a kitten. It amounted to something like, "Oh, that's nice," followed by some weird questions and a quick change of subject. It really hurt. She tried, but she just didn't know what to say.

But many other people did. Though one misses the physical, emotional, and social experience of pregnancy, the adoption process brings with it many other exciting experiences. When we were waiting for my son to come home, my husband shared the news that we were adopting with a man from church, and he gave such a fabulous response. The man said, "Wow, congratulations, and welcome to a very exclusive subset of the parent club." I have found the adoption community to be very supportive and unique. My mother and two of my best friends adopted their children, and we share a connection with one another that my other friends think is really cool, but do not understand from the inside.

Adopting your child is an extraordinary experience. It has so many daunting yet exciting aspects: filling out that first application, preparing your referrals, digging your way out from under the next stack of paperwork, preparing for your home study when you meet and speak with your social worker. My house has never been so clean since that first home study! And then, perhaps after lots more paperwork, you wait anxiously for "the call." I nearly had a panic attack every time the phone rang when I knew "the call" would be coming soon.

The entire time you are waiting you can pray for your child's birthparents, imagine the birthmother discovering her pregnancy, wondering what to do, finally making the hardest and most loving decision of her life, one that will ultimately result in you becoming a parent. As you wait for your child to come home, you can entrust him or her to the care of Jesus and the Blessed Mother. And you can still enjoy the fun of registering for baby shower presents and decorating the nursery if you wish. An incredible rush of emotions will flood over you as you make the final preparations for your child to come home. You may rush to the airport if your child travels to you, or have an incredibly exciting trip if you travel to adopt your child. Or you may get the opportunity to rush to the hospital to bring your child home only days after birth.

Because we were already comfortable with adoption and knew how long it could take, we began exploring it as an option about one month after we decided to stop trying to conceive. Some people would say that was too fast, but it was the right amount of time for us. Some people may prefer to take more time. Others may pursue adoption and biological parenthood simultaneously, willing to try both in the hope that one will succeed. The right amount of time you should take in between stopping fertility treatments and deciding to adopt is up to you; no one else can decide for you. You and your spouse know if you are being honest with God, with yourselves, and with one another. As long as you are both sure that you are being called to adopt and have spent time in prayer about it, by all means move ahead.

The first thing you will realize is that there are many different ways to adopt. My best advice is to read, research, and attend information seminars at various adoption agencies, even if you don't plan to use one. I really liked the book *The Call to Adoption: Becoming Your Child's Family* by Jaymie Stuart Wolfe. It is the only book about adoption I know of that is written from a Catholic perspective, and it is a very good introduction to adoption for those who are beginning to consider it. I also benefitted from talking to other couples who either had adopted already or were considering adoption. The best advice I received was to imagine what I want my future family to look like, and prioritize accordingly. What were my most important considerations as I discerned adopting a child: age? health? race? ethnicity? gender? type of care received prior to placement? cost of adoption? time frame? reliability of the process? degree of openness? amount of preparation provided to adoptive parents (i.e., do you need your hand to be held through the process?)? Answering these questions narrowed down our search considerably and led us to the agency we used and the program that we chose.

The two main ways to adopt a child are domestic adoption and intercountry adoption.[2] Domestic adoption covers both newborn adoption and adoption through public social services. Half of all domestic newborn adoptions in the United States are facilitated through an adoption agency and are called "agency adoption," and the other half are facilitated through an attorney and are called "private adoption" or "identified adoption." Though these two approaches have some differences, they both follow the same basic pattern. After contacting an agency or attorney, prospective adoptive parents complete a home study and draw up a profile of themselves for potential birthparents. In most cases, the birthmother chooses the profile of the couple with whom she wishes to place her child for adoption. However, sometimes agencies or lawyers do the matching. Most domestic adoptions are "open" to some extent. This means that, after substantial preparation, the birthmother and adoptive parents agree to some form of contact after the child is placed for adoption. This contact can be direct or through a third party, and it can range from a picture in the mail once a year to occasional visits, whatever the parties agree upon. The average time frame for domestic newborn adoption varies widely, lasting anywhere from six months to two years.

The Catholic Church has its own adoption programs that are run through Catholic Charities, and they are definitely worth checking out. The average cost of a domestic newborn adoption also varies widely, usually ranging from $27,000 to $35,000. A few agencies, like Catholic Charities, operate on a sliding fee scale and may be significantly less expensive than this range suggests.

Another type of domestic adoption is through the public foster care system. After you qualify, you would receive training and support through your state agency. If you are adopting a child whose biological parents' rights have already been terminated, the adoption proceeds. If you are "fost-adopting" —fostering a child in the hope of adopting him or her once the biological parents' rights have been terminated—your journey begins when you receive the placement of your foster child. It is a difficult yet rewarding task to adopt through the public system, and it is a very popular option. In 2008 the public system handled 55,000 adoptions, almost double the number of domestic newborn adoptions. The age of children adopted through the public system varies widely, though the average age is six years old. The waiting time from placement to adoption also varies widely, and the cost ranges from $0 to $10,000.

Intercountry adoption is another popular way to build your family. Each country has its own set of criteria that prospective parents must meet, so you should check these out before you get your heart set on a particular country's program. According to statistics reported by the Office of

Children's Issues at the United States Department of State, in 2009 the five most popular sending countries, in order of popularity, were China, Ethiopia, Russia, South Korea, and Ukraine. Other popular countries are Vietnam, Haiti, India, Columbia, Philippines, and Taiwan. In most cases, if you qualify for a specific country, you complete a home study and then compile a dossier. This huge stack of paperwork takes a while to gather, and each country has its own specific requirements. Once this is sent to your sending country, you usually wait for the referral of a child (or sometimes you are matched after you travel there). The process varies from one country to the next, but basically after the match is accepted, immigration paperwork needs to be processed and approved by your home country's government, and emigration paperwork needs to be processed and approved by the sending country's government. Then travel arrangements are usually made. Travel requirements vary from no travel required to a stay of four to eight weeks. Some countries require two separate trips by adoptive parents. Sometimes adoptions are legally finalized in the sending country, and sometimes they are legally finalized in the adoptive parents' home country. The cost of international adoption varies widely from agency to agency and country to country. A reliable source of information about adopting from a specific country is an agency that has a history of facilitating adoptions in that country.

If you choose to build your family through adoption, you will digest this information just as you digested all the medical information about infertility. Though it may seem overwhelming at first, you can become an expert on your particular adoption process. You can find so many resources and supportive adoption communities online that there is no reason to undertake this alone. I was amazed at how straightforward our adoption journeys were. The paperwork was tremendous but doable, and we had a wonderful agency and a very supportive caseworker. We joyfully brought our oldest son, and three years later our daughter, home from Korea and into our family forever. We didn't hit one bump in the road in either adoption. In our case, adoption was so much easier than pregnancy. However you become a parent, when you hold your child in your arms, you realize that it was all worth it.

After six years of unexplained infertility, God called my parents to adopt my brother. Five years later they adopted my oldest sister. Though this is the exception and not the rule, five years later they conceived my next oldest sister, and I came along only a year and a half later, quite unexpectedly. Though people will tell you this happens all the time ("Oh watch, as soon as you adopt you'll get pregnant"), it doesn't. The percentage of people who conceive unexpectedly after choosing to adopt is the same as those who do so after choosing to live as a family of two.[3] This myth that adoption helps infertile couples conceive indirectly blames adoptive parents' infertility on their nerves and—hopefully unintentionally—casts their adopted child as a means to conceive a biological child. Though the myth persists and you may hear it if you choose to adopt, adoption does not increase the likelihood that you will conceive a biological child.

Adoption is a beautiful way to build a family. I always knew that my parents had adopted my oldest brother and sister. Adoption was a non-issue for my family. I knew other adopted children, including my best friend and her brother, and I thought all parents adopted at least some of their children. When I found out that this was not the case, I thought those that didn't had missed out on something. When I was about twelve years old, my sister's birthmother initiated contact with her (she was eighteen). I witnessed their beautiful relationship unfold, and was actually jealous of the extra birthday presents she began to receive! My sister was also blessed in getting to know her two younger biological brothers, whom her birthmother was able to parent. In some ways these two young men and their mother have become members of our extended family, loved by us because they gave us our sister and because they are loved by her. They are her family, so they are our family.

Discerning Becoming a Foster Parent

Many couples for whom adoption is not an option still wish to become parents in some way. They still have a deep desire in their hearts to raise and love children, and they may need to consider if God is calling them to become foster parents. So many children are waiting to receive the stability of a loving mother and father and a nurturing home. When children's biological parents cannot care for them yet still retain legal parental rights, foster parents are needed. They can give these sweet angels a chance to know what it is to be loved and cared for by a mother and father who can see to their physical, emotional, and spiritual needs until their biological parents can care for them again.

Foster care programs place children in the temporary care of foster parents. The civil authorities can remove children from their biological parents' care for many reasons, including but not limited to abuse and neglect. As with adoption, becoming foster parents does not cure infertility; it temporarily cures childlessness. Becoming a foster parent will not fulfill your desire to experience pregnancy, nor will it completely fulfill your desire to permanently and legally become a parent to a child (unless you are able to adopt your foster child). Unlike adoption, foster parenting is not permanent. By its very nature, foster care is meant to be a temporary solution to a temporary problem that will hopefully be permanently resolved in a way that allows foster children to be reunited with their biological parents. Though some foster children become available for adoption, as was discussed earlier, most foster children's biological parents are following a plan given to them by their social workers to ultimately regain custody of their children.

So, becoming a foster parent means that you are temporarily parenting a child with the ultimate goal of preparing that child to be reunited with their permanent family. This means that your generous love for your foster children must be without limits, even as you go into each relationship with each foster child knowing that he or she will not be yours forever. You cannot hold back love, yet you need to be prepared—and you need to prepare your foster child—for the day when the child will be placed back in the care of the biological parents. It is a tremendously difficult yet unbelievably rewarding calling, and if God has foster parenting in mind for you, he will give you everything you need to do it. I know foster parents who are still visited by their now grown foster children, who still affectionately call them Mom and Dad. Foster parenting asks you to give a piece of your heart to all of your foster children. But instead of having no pieces left, God constantly enlarges your heart so you have more to give.

Both of our adopted children were cared for by wonderful foster parents before they came to us. After their birth parents made adoption plans for them, my oldest son and my daughter were placed with loving foster families until their adoption and immigration paperwork went through. These families loved my children as if they were their own. They cared for them with tremendous generosity and selflessness. Foster parenting isn't babysitting—it's parenting!

I had the privilege of meeting my children's foster parents, and I saw the love and pain in their eyes as they placed their children—now my children—in my arms. Both of the couples who were foster parents for my children continued to foster other children who awaited their forever families. It is their calling. Pictures of them holding my children will always be on the bookshelf in my living room, next to other important family pictures. I'm sure they have pictures of my children in their homes as well. My children know their names and ask about them. We send them letters and pictures so they can see how their foster children—my children—are growing and blossoming.

When we went to Korea a second time to bring our daughter home, our son's foster parents came to the agency to see us again. They had a small gift for my son, and we both cried upon seeing each other as if they were relinquishing my son all over again. They miss him terribly, as I'm sure my daughter's foster parents do. Their love and sacrifices made it possible for my son and daughter to come home to us, and we are forever grateful.

Discerning a Family of Two

For many couples who struggle with infertility, adoption and foster parenting are simply not options. The many reasons for this include but are not limited to financial, medical, emotional, or personal factors. A couple may not feel drawn to adoption or foster parenting at all. Whatever their reasons, they need to be respected and not questioned. Just as infertile couples may choose to keep the reasons for their infertility to themselves, couples who are unable or who choose not to adopt or become foster parents may also wish to keep their reasons private. When these couples decide to stop trying to conceive, the possibility of becoming parents comes to an end.

The decision to not bring children into your family is a difficult one to make, especially for Catholics because our vocation to marriage places us at the service of life. Consequently, much of our Church seems to be built around children. Most churches are built with additional space for religious education programs or schools for children. As Catholics, whenever we hear the word "family," we immediately imagine a mother, a father, and any number of children (traditionally, the more the merrier).

But this image is not the only one possible. A man and a woman become a family as soon as they exchange their marriage vows. Though at our wedding liturgy we promised to be open to having children and to raise them in our faith, this does not mean that couples who struggle with infertility are required to adopt or become foster parents. Children are a gift to be received, not a right to be demanded. Certainly if a husband and wife cannot conceive a child, they are free to embrace life as a family of two. The meaning of their marriage is not lessened in any way in the eyes of God or the Church. Every mention of children in the ritual for the sacrament of marriage is in parentheses, so these can be omitted in cases where it is already known that the spouses cannot conceive or if the couple is advanced in years.[4]

Our faith is reflected in how we celebrate our most sacred rituals. Marriage retains its meaning and value as a good unto itself, even when spouses cannot conceive through no fault of their own. The *Catechism of the Catholic Church* states: "Spouses to whom God has not granted children can nevertheless have a conjugal life full of meaning, in both human and Christian terms. Their marriage can radiate a fruitfulness of charity, of hospitality, and of sacrifice."[5] Spouses who choose to end their pursuit of parenthood have not changed their vocation. God called them to be true to one another and honor each other all the days of their lives no matter the cost. Not having children does not change that. God calls all spouses, not just those who happen to be parents, to make a sincere gift of sacrificial love to one another and to others. It is precisely in this way that all married couples reflect God's love to the world. This self-giving, sacrificial love is the crowning glory of married life, regardless of whether or not children are at the receiving end.

How, then, is this love to be lived out? This question must be answered by couples who decide to end their pursuit of parenthood. Catholics can live out their vocation to sacrificial love as a family of two in any number of ways. Each couple is unique. Many choose to involve themselves with children, either in their work or on a volunteer basis. Others dedicate themselves to improving the lives of the needy. Though all Catholics are called to do this, those who do not have children can do this in a much different way.

When we are going through the pain of infertility, we may tend to romanticize parenthood and fantasize about it in an unrealistic way. But we have to realize the constraints of parenthood. As a Catholic mother, God is my first priority, my marriage is my second priority, and my children are my third priority. Keeping these priorities in order is a challenge when a diaper needs to be changed, a math problem needs to be worked out, a second spill needs to be cleaned up, a favorite toy needs to be found, the mountain of laundry needs to be put away—and it's only nine o'clock in the morning. Preparing lunch for five isn't even on my radar yet—let alone dinner—and so far I'm sizing it up to be a pretty light day! It is a constant challenge to carve out time to pray and deepen my relationship with God and also to make time to enjoy and strengthen my marriage.

On an average day, my children receive well over half of my time and energy. I'd love to do so many things—go on a spiritual retreat, do volunteer work at church, and take a vacation with my husband. On many days I long for the spiritual depth lived out by cloistered nuns whose prayer is their work and whose work is their prayer. I often feel neglectful of my relationships with family and friends, especially those with my girlfriends who do not have young children. If you can't meet me at a park and have a conversation with me that is constantly interrupted by kissing scraped knees, breaking up arguments, and searching for the "flight risk" child who likes to hide in public places, I may not get to talk to you for some time. That is simply the reality of motherhood for me at this stage of my family's growth.

God has called me to parenthood, and though these other pursuits are worthy and certainly pleasing to God, they are not possible for me right now. Some will have to wait, and some will never happen. I don't begrudge this, either. It is simply the life that I have been called to, the life that God has chosen me for, the path that God desires to use to bring me to eternal life with him in heaven. Life as a family of two is simply another path, another way to live out one's vocation to married life, another call that God can use to bring couples into union with him.

More than anything else, Catholics who are a family of two have the gift of time. As with the journey through infertility, this brings almost limitless choices for spouses to make. How will they spend their time? It calls for serious discernment of one's talents, gifts, interests, and resources. Life as a family of two is not a call to "childlessness," which focuses on what a couple is not called to. It is a definite call to love and life-giving service to the Church and to the world. Each couple with this distinctive call must prayerfully discern the particular path God desires them to take. The needs of the Church and the world are as many and varied as the gifts, talents, and interests of those couples whose marriage and family life offer them the flexibility and availability to meet these needs.

> A profound unity exists between the soul and the body. They are not two separate natures joined together in the human person, but rather they are an integrated union that forms a single nature . . . Our entire being is meant to be life-giving, life-producing. Our call to bring life to others, then, does not stop at the physical level, but only begins there . . . our call to motherhood is in no way diminished or negated by . . . an inability to physically bear children. *All women are meant to bring life.*[6]

Though the above statement is directed to women, it is also true for men. I like to think of the call to life as a family of two in the context of vocation and one's state in life. Our fundamental Christian vocation is rooted in Baptism. All the baptized are called to holiness and to share in Christ's mission. God calls certain men in the Church to the vocation of holy orders as deacons, priests, and bishops. God calls other men and women to consecrated life as sisters, nuns, brothers, and monks. And finally, God calls most other members of the lay faithful to the vocation of marriage. However, some members of the laity live out their baptismal call to holiness in the context of single life. Each of these ways is a gift from God for the person who receives it. In all of these states of life, we are called to be in life-giving relationship with others, to care for our Church and our world. We are all called to make a sincere gift of self and unite ourselves with Jesus's cross in order to bring forth life.

While most people in the Church are called to married life, and most of those in married life are called to parenthood, most clergy, religious, and single people are not called to parenthood. They all figure out how to have happy and deeply meaningful lives outside of parenthood. Besides nurturing their relationships with God and one another, couples who do not have children can look to their counterparts in other states of life for ideas on how to live out their call to life-giving service. Their first priority will always be their relationship with God (as is true for all Catholics), and their second priority will always be their relationship with their spouse (as is true for all married Catholics). What is their third priority? It could be their career, volunteer work, elderly parents, nieces and nephews, helping the poor, joining service organizations, or even becoming missionaries. Discovering the answer to this question brings countless possibilities! It is time to dream new dreams and search your heart for the place where your deepest desires meet the world's deepest needs. That is your third priority. That is the path God has called you to follow as a family of two. That is your life's work, and it is a gift from God to be embraced with joy.

Bearing Fruit in the Desert

Led by the Spirit of God into the desert, Christ fasted and prayed for forty days to prepare himself to carry out his mission from God the Father. In the desert, Christ suffered physical hunger, battled temptation, and depended utterly on the Father to meet his every need. After Jesus came out of the desert, he began his public life, inviting others to repent and believe in the Gospel.

Jesus said that following him would involve picking up our cross each day. Infertility is a distinctive journey some of us are called to travel, and though it brings great suffering, God can use it to bear great fruit in our lives. If my parents were not infertile, they would not have adopted my brother and sister. If my husband and I were not infertile, we would not have adopted our oldest son and daughter. I also would not have my second son, who came to us through an unexpected and quite miraculous pregnancy. As the mommy to these three precious angels, I dare not even contemplate life without each one of them.

Through infertility, God has also enriched our lives with Korean culture and given me two of my best friends, who also adopted their children from South Korea and have preserved my sanity on more than one occasion. God also led my husband and me down a path in our lives that allowed us to host a high school exchange student from South Korea, who is now like a daughter to us. She decided to become Catholic, and is now my goddaughter. Though she now lives in South Korea with her parents again, she knows she always has a home with us. We continue to be in touch with her across the ocean. All of these wonderful, life-giving relationships blossomed because God enabled us to use our infertility to bring about great fruit in our lives and in the lives of others.

God also used infertility to strengthen my marriage and my relationships with my parents, brother, and sisters. When God gave me the will to reclaim my body from infertility and lose the weight that I had gained because of grief, he brought me to a place of physical health and confidence I may never have known otherwise. He changed my life forever. I am the person I am now because God raised me from the death that infertility dealt me. Infertility forced me to find new ways to be fruitful, and I directed my creative energy into cooking, a therapeutic (and useful) hobby without which I may have gone mad many times over. I am now a confessed cooking addict and foodie, and can't imagine my life without my kitchen. (I know my husband would also count this as a blessing.)

I probably never would have studied Tae Kwon Do or taken up running if we had initially been able to conceive. It has been such a blessing to realize that even though I couldn't get pregnant, physically I could do some other spectacular things. Infertility caused a disconnect between my inner self and my body, like the two were at war. Many women share this experience. For me, healthy physical activity brought me back into my body in many ways and made me a healthier person.

Because of my infertility, I was moved to ask the diocese where I worked as a chaplain to initiate an adoption benefits program, through which it became the first Catholic diocese in the United States to offer financial assistance and paid leave to its employees who build their family through adoption. Through my infertility, God placed it on my heart to initiate a Catholic ministry to couples struggling with infertility. And I felt called by God to write this book, which has been a very fruitful experience for me, in the hope that it will bear great fruit in your life as well.

In short, God has used infertility to make me into the person I am today, which I think is closer to the person he created me to be than the person I was before. He has completely re-created me by allowing me to suffer the pain of being infertile. And on this side of the experience, I can honestly say without the slightest hesitation that I am truly grateful to God for the fruitfulness that the cross of infertility has brought.

Like Jesus, the desert that has closed in upon us has called us to great suffering, longing, and radical dependence on God. It has given us an opportunity to allow God to clarify for us what he desires for us and from us. Infertility brought each one of us into this desert experience, but God has walked beside us through our entire journey. If we remain in his presence and love, he will enable us to bear great fruit in our lives. That fruit may or may not include biological children, adopted children, foster children, or life as a family of two. Whatever future God has in mind for us, it is better than anything we can possibly imagine. Walking into that future with him, depending on him to tell us what the next move should be, will teach us to trust him. That trust in him has tremendous value, and is the most important fruit we bear in the desert. In fact, that radical trust in him and utter abandonment to his will is the only way out of the desert.

QUESTIONS FOR REFLECTION AND DISCUSSION

ᴥ Can you imagine you or your spouse ever discerning a call to adoption? If so, what are your concerns, fears, or questions?

- ❧ If you are willing to discern a call to adoption, what are your most important considerations: age, health, race, ethnicity, or gender of the child? The type of care the child received prior to placement? The cost of adoption? The timeframe, reliability of the process, or its degree of openness? The amount of preparation provided to adoptive parents?

- ❧ Can you imagine you or your spouse ever discerning a call to foster parenting? If so, what are your concerns, fears, or questions?

- ❧ Can you imagine you and your spouse ever discerning a call to a family of two as a possibility? If so, what are your concerns, fears, or questions?

- ❧ Can you identify any ways in which God has used your infertility to bring about good in your life or in the lives of others?

- ❧ What would you like to share with your spouse from your reflection?

For Family and Friends

Learning that your loved ones are considering alternatives to biological parenthood may bring relief or disappointment. As difficult as it may be, it will help them if you try to stay with them in their experience, not lagging too far behind or getting too far ahead of them. Yes, their decisions will impact your life in some way, especially if you are their parent. But you must try to trust in God's will for their lives just as they are hopefully learning to trust him. More than anything else, a positive attitude of openness and sensitivity on your part will go a long way to providing them with the support they need to move into their future.

Prayer

Protect me, O God, for in you I take refuge.
I say to the Lord, *"You are my Lord;*
   I have no good apart from you." . . .
The Lord *is my chosen portion and my cup;*
   you hold my lot.
The boundary lines have fallen for me in pleasant places;
   I have a goodly heritage.
I bless the Lord *who gives me counsel;*
   in the night also my heart instructs me.
I keep the Lord *always before me;*
   because he is at my right hand, I shall not be moved.
Therefore my heart is glad, and my soul rejoices;
   my body also rests secure. . . .
You show me the path of life.
   In your presence there is fullness of joy;
   in your right hand are pleasures forevermore.

Psalm 16:1–2, 5–9, 11

Chapter 10

Following God
in the Midst of Suffering

My God, my God, why have you forsaken me?
Why are you so far from helping me, from the words
of my groaning?
O my God, I cry by day, but you do not answer;
and by night, but find no rest.

PSALM 22:1–2

We are technically not infertile. We have conceived seven times. Six pregnancies ended in miscarriage, and one with a stillbirth.[1] After our first child died at twenty-seven weeks, I was angry at God. I still loved God and went to church, but I stopped praying for the gift of a child. I thought, *What good is it to pray for something when God knows how it will turn out anyway? When I prayed so hard my little girl died anyway.* It was a tough place to be in my relationship with

God. I believed in him with my whole heart but thought he didn't love me. I felt alone and abandoned, like a small life in his big scheme of things.

I've grown to know that he does love me unconditionally. I think we live in a broken world. Life is not pain free; things are not fair. God made it possible for us to adopt. We are blessed to have our son. I think God is good. He put us, two people who desperately wanted a child, together with our son, a child who desperately needed parents. How perfect is that?

— T. E.

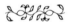

Why Me, Lord?

Many couples who experience the pain of infertility begin to question their relationship with God. Some may even begin to feel abandoned by God and blame him for their condition. It is difficult to understand how an all-powerful God who loves us unconditionally could allow this to happen. They may wonder if they are being punished for some reason, perhaps even believing that God doesn't want them to be parents. Although couples struggling with infertility often have such thoughts and feelings, they represent a fundamental misunderstanding about God and about the source of human suffering. While it is tempting to believe that since God is all-powerful, everything that happens to us in life must be his doing, this is absolutely not the case.

Our Catholic faith teaches us that God is the author of goodness, beauty, life, and love. We read in the first chapter of Genesis that God looked at everything he had created and saw that it was good. God works to bring about only good. God does not create suffering and death. God never directly wills anything of the sort. Evil, in fact, is the lack of a good that ought to be present.

God desires only the fullness of life for his people, as he has from all eternity. God created humankind with free will so that it might always have a peaceful relationship with God, one another, and the created world. In the Garden of Eden, Adam and Eve experienced no pain, sorrow, or death. We all know the story of flowing rivers, blossoming vegetation, peaceful creatures, immortality, and companionship with a perfect spouse and with God (see Gen 1 and 2).

But in the third chapter of Genesis, sin comes into play. Here we encounter the mystery of the fallen state of humanity. Though they had everything they could possibly need for true and lasting happiness, our first parents freely and intentionally chose to disobey God. Adam and Eve did exactly what God told them not to do and ate fruit from the one tree that was forbidden to them. Believing the lie of the serpent, they sacrificed true and eternal human happiness—the life God intended for all of us—because of their desire to be like God.

This story of our human origins lays the foundation for what Catholics refer to as original sin. The *Catechism* explains: "It is a sin which will be transmitted by propagation to all mankind, that is, by the transmission of a human nature deprived of original holiness and justice. And that is why original sin is called 'sin' only in an analogical sense: it is a sin 'contracted' and not 'committed'—a state and not an act."[2]

Because of this first sin, suffering and death entered human experience and play a role in the life of every human being.

This theological trek into the Book of Genesis is not meant to be some kind of vague Sunday school lesson. It is meant to explain how God's originally perfect world came to be imperfect, and that it is not God's doing. I would like to stress that:

God did not create infertility.

God never punishes anyone with infertility.

God does not desire infertility for any of us.

God made us and all of creation flawless, and sin has disfigured us. All forms of human suffering—including infertility—are the result of original sin. If we feel we must blame someone or something for our infertility, we can blame human sinfulness. We cannot, however, blame God. God loves us unconditionally and he has intervened throughout human history to heal and redeem us.

Infertility indeed raises profound questions, but it is certainly not a punishment from a remote, heartless deity. It is not supposed to happen at all. It is solely the result of one or more things going wrong with the human reproductive system. This system is delicate and intricate, and even in cases of unexplained infertility, something has physically gone wrong in some way. Why does this happen? There is no satisfying explanation. Like other physical diseases and disabilities, infertility occurs because we live in an imperfect world.

> But with infinite wisdom and goodness God freely willed to create a world 'in a state of journeying' toward its ultimate perfection. In God's plan this process of becoming involves . . . the existence of the more perfect alongside the less perfect, both constructive and destructive forces of nature. With physical good there exists also *physical* evil as long as creation has not reached perfection.[3]

Original sin has disfigured all of creation, including us. But in his great love for us, God sent his Son Jesus Christ to meet us in the desert of our fallen humanity and lead us to salvation, so that we may have the opportunity to be who God created us to be and live forever in eternal happiness with him.

Lost in the Desert

The word "desert" comes from the Latin "dēsertum," which means "an abandoned place." Infertility is exactly this. In a desert, it is easy to get lost and to feel abandoned. Navigation during the day is difficult, and navigation at night requires an intimate knowledge of the stars. Desert travelers have been known to die while wandering in circles, only miles away from a well that could have saved their life. The only safe way to travel through the desert is with an experienced guide.

When the Israelites wandered through the desert for forty years after their exodus from slavery in Egypt, they felt abandoned by God. They felt lost and alone in an unfamiliar land with nothing to drink or eat. Yet God did not leave them. He appeared to them as a pillar of cloud by day and a pillar of fire by night, leading them through the desert (see Ex 13). God also miraculously provided the Israelites with water from a rock and manna from heaven, which they made into bread (see Ex 16 and 17). This heavenly food and drink preserved their lives until they reached the Promised Land.

Like our ancestors the Israelites, we who experience infertility can also feel lost and alone, as if God has abandoned us. We hunger and thirst for a child like the Israelites hungered and thirsted in the desert. Our desire for a child is so strong that sometimes we feel like Rachel and cry out to God, "Give me children, or I shall die!" (Gen 30:1). The searing pain of infertility threatens to completely unravel our lives. Yet God will never leave us. *He loves us and longs for us even more than we long for a child.* When we feel utterly forsaken by God, he says to us: "Can a woman forget her nursing child, or show no compassion for the child of her womb? Even these may forget, yet I will not forget you. . . . Then you will know that I am the Lord; those who wait for me shall not be put to shame" (Is 49:15, 23b).

God is our Father. He created us and loves us. He is faithful and will never abandon us. Whether or not we have been aware of his presence, God has been with us, loving us unconditionally, at every moment of our lives. He was there when we married. He was there when we first desired to become parents. He was there every time we tried to conceive, and he was there as we read the results of every pregnancy test. God was there at the beginning of every month of our cycle when we realized we were not pregnant. He was there when our doctors told us our diagnosis. He was there when our pregnancy ended in the horror of miscarriage. God has always been with us, loving us and reaching out to us. He is with us at this very moment, loving us and desiring to lead us into our future.

God gave the Israelites water from a rock and manna from heaven. What does God give to us to preserve our lives as we hunger and thirst for a child in this desert? He gives us his Son, Jesus Christ.

Saint Paul tells us that when God gave the Israelites water from the rock, the water was really Christ (see 1 Cor 10:4). Our Lord tells us that the Eucharist, his Body and Blood, is real food and drink sent down from heaven to give us life (see Jn 6:48–51). Jesus himself is our guide and our nourishment in the desert. He wants us to be as madly in love with him as he is with us. *He loves us and longs for us even more than we long for a child.* When we receive Jesus in the Eucharist, we are enveloped in his love for us. He loves us so much that he died for us, so that we could be with him forever. He has already traveled the road of grief and loss, and he knows the path that lies ahead of us. He can see far above the storm raging about us, and he alone can lead us through it to the land where the desert ends.

Lord of the Desert

We have many good reasons to trust Jesus to lead us through the pain of our infertility, and two in particular that I find compelling. First, Jesus loves us unconditionally; and second, he has already suffered grief and loss through his own death, so he understands our suffering completely. As we endure our own pain and grief, we can learn to imitate Jesus as he suffered for us. Jesus, the Son of God, proclaimed the coming of the kingdom of God and called people to turn away from sin and return to an intimate relationship with God. Jesus performed many miracles, healed many sick people, and gathered and taught a community of followers. His teachings and ministry caught the attention of the religious and political leaders of his day, and they ultimately sentenced him to death by crucifixion.

Catholics refer to the events leading up to his death as the Passion of Christ. The word "passion" comes from the Greek "*paschō*," which means "I suffer." Anticipating his own suffering and death, Jesus prepared his followers for it. On the night before he died, Jesus shared the Eucharist with his disciples, instituting this meal as a perpetual sacrifice, forever giving his Church a means to receive the grace of salvation that he won for us when he died and rose. After supper, Jesus and his disciples went to the Garden of Gethsemane, where Jesus began to show signs of the depths of his suffering.

In his humanity, Jesus experienced deep movements of grief and pain, similar to our own. As he prayed in the garden, he was abandoned by his friends, who had no idea what he was going through. Even his closest friends, Peter, James, and John, were so emotionally exhausted that they could not even stay awake to keep watch with him through the night. Can't we all relate to his experience? Even our closest friends, possibly even our spouses, sometimes have no idea how to support us in our suffering. We often find ourselves completely alone with Jesus in our own garden of agony.

Then Jesus fell to the ground and prayed intensely, begging to be rescued from death: "Abba, Father, for you all things are possible; remove this cup from me; yet, not what I want, but what you want" (Mk 14:36). How many hours have we spent begging God to take away our suffering? Jesus didn't relish the idea of physical suffering. On the contrary, he begged God to protect him from it. But because he was confident in his Father's love for him, though he said, "I am deeply grieved, even to death" (Mt 26:38), Jesus was still willing to accept his Father's response. Should we not also pray for the grace of such a willing spirit, ready to follow wherever God leads?

Jesus knew that he was going to be betrayed, denied, tortured, and murdered. In the Garden of Gethsemane, Jesus saw in his future unfathomable pain and suffering. Yet instead of relying on his own human understanding, he trusted his future to his Father. Isn't that fortunate for us, the benefactors of Jesus's act of redemption? What wonderful things God can do when we follow him, no matter the cost. In the same way, God can use our present suffering to bring about greater good for our lives if we let him, even though we do not fully comprehend it now.

Jesus knows our loneliness and our desire to escape suffering. He also knows the depths of our sadness. He is with us now, loving us, waiting for us to surrender our suffering to him and abandon ourselves to his healing embrace. If we seek his will, he can lead us safely through the desert until we reach its end.

Though Jesus obediently gave up his life out of love for us, he suffered greatly. He was beaten and bruised, embarrassed and shamed, and stripped of all dignity. The aesthetically pleasing crucifix hanging in church belies the fact that Jesus died bloody, broken, and naked, for all to see. How similar is our experience of infertility? How many times have we been stripped of all our clothes save a hospital gown? How many times have we been poked and prodded, on display for doctors and nurses to examine? How many times have our bodies been ravaged by surgery and fertility drugs? Even the most superficial fertility tests and treatments can expose our most intimate moments with our spouse to clinical testing, embarrassing questions, and demeaning scrutiny. With Christ, we all have worn a crown of thorns: "And the soldiers wove a crown of thorns and put it on his head, and they dressed him in a purple robe. They kept coming up to him, saying, 'Hail, King of the Jews!' and striking him on the face" (Jn 19:2–3).

Hanging on the cross in the final moments of his life, Jesus called out to God in distress quoting the first few words of Psalm 22, saying, "My God, my God, why have you forsaken me?" (Mt 27:46). Jesus fully understands what it means to feel lost and abandoned by God. However, though the Gospel accounts do not record Jesus reciting the entire psalm, surely Jesus knew that this psalm ends in hope and trust. Jesus knew his Father would never abandon him. Though he was enduring tremendous pain and suffering, Jesus knew that his Father had never left him. Instead, Jesus relied on him for strength as he drew his last breath, trusting his future to his loving Abba even as he was moments from death.

The Catholic Church has a long-standing, venerable idea that may have unfortunately passed over many of us in our religious upbringing—the concept of redemptive suffering. It is the idea that though human suffering is a horrible thing, and though God does not cause human suffering, we can and should allow God to use it to bring about good while we are going through it. This idea may never win any popularity contests, since most of us will try to avoid suffering if we can. But for the times in life when we cannot avoid it, we can offer our suffering to God to be united with Christ's unique sacrifice on the cross. As Saint Paul said, "In my flesh I am completing what is lacking in Christ's afflictions for the sake of his body, that is, the church" (Col 1:24). Remember the old phrase "offer it up"? It still applies. That is why Catholics still do penance after we confess our sins and still fast and abstain, especially during Lent when we focus on Christ's passion. Our suffering has redemptive potential, that is, it can bring about good if we allow God to use it for his purposes. Though we will not always see or understand the fruits of our suffering right away (some we will never see at all), we can trust God to bring about the greatest possible good if we give ourselves over to his grace. This is one of the many ways that we can bear fruit in the desert. Of course we would all rather not be in this desert, but since we are here, what good can we allow God to bring forth from us?

Because of his love for us, Jesus suffered and died to remove our guilt, to undo the consequences of original sin, and to offer us the possibility of salvation. Jesus used pain and death to have the final say over sin and evil and open again the way to eternal life. Through his one act of obedience, Jesus undid the disobedience of Adam and Eve.

Because of his love for us, Jesus then rose to new life in the resurrection, becoming a source of healing and grace for those who believe in him. *He loves us and longs for us even more than we long for a child.* If we surrender the suffering of our infertility to Jesus and abandon ourselves to his loving embrace on the cross, we open ourselves up to his healing grace. God has the power to heal us physically, emotionally, and spiritually. It is up to us to ask him for this healing, and to accept it in whatever form it comes.

QUESTIONS FOR REFLECTION AND DISCUSSION

ॐ What effect has your experience of infertility had on your relationship with God? Or what impact has your relationship with God had on your experience of infertility? Please describe.

ॐ After reading this chapter, how do you understand the ultimate cause of your infertility? How can you answer the question, "Why me, Lord?"

ॐ Do you believe that God loves you and longs for you even more than you long for a child? How does that make you feel?

ॐ Remember all the significant moments along your personal journey of infertility, imagining Jesus with you in each of them. Recall his great love for you, and allow him to speak to your heart in prayer as you remember these moments of pain and sorrow.

∞ How does it make you feel to know that Jesus suffered abandonment, that he asked God to take away his suffering, that he said he could die from sorrow, and that he was stripped of all dignity?

∞ Do you think you could pray with Jesus, "Lord not my will, but thy will be done"? What would you need to do in order to make that prayer your own? With the help of God's grace, do you think you could do this and abandon yourself to God and trust your future to him?

∞ If you offer your suffering to God, what good do you think God could bring out of it? What fruit can you bear in this desert?

∞ What would you like to share with your spouse from your reflection?

For Family and Friends

People going through infertility often feel isolated and abandoned, perhaps even by God. Do your best to be a source of emotional support and encouragement. Try to take their suffering as seriously as they do. Try to keep them connected to you and other loved ones. If you can, remind them that Jesus knows exactly what they are going through, that he is with them always and loves them, and that he has a plan already worked out for them.

Prayer

You who live in the shelter of the Most High,
who abide in the shadow of the Almighty,
will say to the Lord, "My refuge and my fortress;
my God, in whom I trust."
For he will deliver you from the snare of the fowler
and from the deadly pestilence;
he will cover you with his pinions,
and under his wings you will find refuge;
his faithfulness is a shield and buckler. . . .
Because you have made the Lord your refuge,
the Most High your dwelling place,
no evil shall befall you,
no scourge come near your tent.

Psalm 91:1–4, 9–10

Chapter 11

Coming to the End of Our Journey

On this mountain the Lord *of hosts will make for*
      all peoples
   a feast of rich food. . . .
      he will swallow up death forever. . . .
For the hand of the Lord *will rest on this mountain.*

Isaiah 25:6, 8, 10

For me, infertility was definitely a faith-growing experience. My husband and I found out while we were still dating that we would probably not be able to conceive. After we married and started trying to get pregnant, we decided we would only try for a few years, and that we wouldn't use assisted reproductive technology. Even though from as far back as I can remember I have always wanted to be pregnant, God showed us that it was more important for us to become parents than it was for us to have a biological child. His will for our lives led us to adoption.

But I will always remember something that happened during my experience of infertility. One night when we were still trying to conceive, I was driving home from Bible study and listening to a Christian radio station. A woman who was talking about her struggle with infertility said that she prayed to love God and to want his will for her life more than she wanted a baby. That thought struck me and remains with me to this day. I clung to that prayer and tried to make it my own. Every day I remind myself that his will for my life is more important than anything else I might want.

— J. T.

A person who sets out on a journey usually has a particular destination in mind. When we first set foot on the path that we had hoped would lead to parenthood, our perceived destination was pregnancy. We did not anticipate that our path would lead us into the desert. Yet that is where we found ourselves. It was not the destination we intended, but it was the one to which God accompanied us.

At first we believed that the desert was only a detour on our otherwise direct route, and we desperately searched for a way out so that we could aim for parenthood once again. We endured our time of suffering here with the hope that we were only passing through, and that pregnancy was just over the next hill. When that hill turned out to be a precipice that sharply dropped off into an abyss, we realized that we would have to allow God to chart a new course for us. We would have to let Jesus guide us through this unfamiliar terrain. Once we did that, our suffering did not end. On the contrary, it was just beginning.

Jesus did not promise his followers an easy road, nor did he guarantee that life would be filled with cheerfulness and pleasure. Instead, he spoke about taking up our cross and following him. Following Jesus means following him on the road to Calvary without counting the cost. "Whoever loves father or mother more than me is not worthy of me; and whoever loves son or daughter more than me is not worthy of me; and whoever does not take up the cross and follow me is not worthy of me. Those who find their life will lose it, and those who lose their life for my sake will find it" (Mt 10:37–39). Thankfully the cross leads to the empty tomb—death eventually leads to resurrection.

These words are very hard to hear for those whose all-consuming desire in life is for the gift of a child. But Jesus will not force us to follow him. Surely, if we desire ultimate fulfillment and happiness in this life and the next, then we must follow him wherever he leads us. If we do, we will be grateful to find the oases in the desert. They are places where we can experience earthly happiness and bounty, wells we can drink from, and communities in which we can thrive. Yet they all exist within the desert of our life experience, and sometimes our path will lead us away from the oases, the wells, and earthly happiness, and into the blinding storms.

As I often returned in prayer to the image of my husband and I clinging to Christ in the desert, blindly bracing ourselves against the storm raging all around us, I began to discern in my mind's eye a distant horizon, a place where the desert meets the sky. Relying on the biblical imagery of the

Israelites in the desert, and of Christ with his disciples on the mount where he was transfigured, I began to imagine a mountain on the horizon. I kept praying to Jesus to lead me to that mountain, desperately hoping he had children for me there. I promised to continue to trust him and follow him, yet I needed to know whether or not he had children in mind for me, and if so, whether they were biological children or adopted children. I didn't know what he wanted me to do, and I mistakenly believed that I needed to know what the final destination was in order to follow him. Yet, the image was too distant, too clouded. I couldn't make it out. I could only sense Jesus relentlessly leading me onward.

As the storm settled down and I realized, as I then believed, that I would not conceive, I redirected my spiritual gaze toward that mountain on the horizon. While I still couldn't see any of its details, Jesus made it quite clear to me that my husband and I would not reach it alone. While our eyes were still fixed on our ultimate destination, our children suddenly joined us in our walk with Christ and began to journey with us through the desert. First came our faithful angel John, quickly followed by our hope-filled treasure Joseph, and, most recently, our loving joy Lucianna. I've come to realize that the desert never ends in this life, and that Christ our guide is ultimately leading us, not to parenthood, but to eternal life with him. The mountain on the horizon, that place in the hazy distance where the sand meets the sky, is not parenthood, but heaven itself.

Infertility is a part of our whole life's journey to God. It will eventually yield either a family grown through pregnancy, adoption, and/or foster parenting, or life as a family of two. Whichever of these paths God lays out for us, they will all lead to the same place as long as we continue to follow his Son. The grace of marriage, lived out in a family with children or in a family of two, is a means to an end. Parenthood is not an end unto itself, and neither is marriage. Rather, they are distinct paths on which God leads us to bring us to the ultimate reason for our existence: eternal life with him in heaven.

Whether we knew it or not, we began our life's journey in the desert that is the human condition. Even before we were conceived in our mother's womb, God had a plan for each of us. The deepest desire of God's heart is for us to freely choose to be in an intimate and eternal union of love with him. That is why he created us as embodied spirits. We are not merely physical creatures, doomed to die and never live again. Nor are we angels of pure spirit. We are fully human persons, whose bodies are destined to die and be raised up, joined to immortal souls bound for eternity. God designed us to long for him. We are built for relationship with him. This yearning of our hearts for God is his plan for the human person, intended to lead us back to him. Nothing that life can give us, not even children, will ever truly satisfy the deep craving of our hearts. God made us in his image and likeness, an act of creative love spilling out of the Love that is Father, Son, and Holy Spirit.

So why did God make us? To be parents? No. To be married? No. Then why? If you ask your parents or grandparents, they may remember the answer they learned as children as it was presented in the *Baltimore Catechism*. The simple, yet profound answer found there is this: "God made us to show forth his goodness and to share with us his everlasting happiness in heaven."[1] All other priorities in life, worthy though they may be, fall in line after this one.

Parenthood has made me a more mature Catholic, given me a much broader perspective than I previously had, and tremendously deepened my relationship with Christ. I am still woefully far from being the person God created me to be, so I still have plenty more work to do, but I believe I'm a little farther along than I was before. Jesus has continued to teach me over and over that his love and longing for me are greater than my love and longing for my children. When my husband and I were going through infertility, I thought that my ultimate destination in life, the holy mountain where the desert ends, was motherhood. Now I know this to be false. Rather, motherhood is one of the ways Christ uses to bring me to my true ultimate destination: eternal life with him. Had I never become a mother, God would have given me another path that would lead to eternity with him. If I am not a mother, then who am I? Even if I am a mother, who am I *really*? I am a child of God, designed for eternal life in intimate relationship with him. Though I may wish at times to be many other things, that is all I really ever need to be.

QUESTIONS FOR REFLECTION AND DISCUSSION

- ✽ Describe your reaction to the following statement: "Parenthood is not an end unto itself."

- ✽ Can you bring yourself to imagine that there might be an ultimate goal in your life more important than parenthood? If so, how would you describe that goal?

- ✽ Do you think that re-orienting yourself on the path that leads to eternal life with God and directing your gaze there would adjust your perspective on your infertility? If so, how?

- ✽ Even if you never become a parent, who do you believe yourself to be at the innermost core of your being?

∞ What would you like to share with your spouse from your reflection?

For Family and Friends

The desire for children can become an all-consuming mission for those who struggle with infertility. The quest for pregnancy can overshadow so many other aspects of a person's life, and may sometimes bring about a loss of perspective. As you journey with your loved ones, do your best to be emotionally available to them, reflecting their feelings back to them and letting them know that they are heard. At the same time, try to bring a sense of perspective to help your loved ones refocus, if you can do that in a sensitive way that they can hear and receive. If you know someone else who needs prayers, ask your loved one to pray for them. Sometimes focusing on other people's needs helps remind us of how blessed we are. Ultimately, be prepared to let them teach you exactly what it is that they need from you to help them through their experience.

Prayer
(Canticle of Simeon)

"Master, now you are dismissing your servant in peace,
*   according to your word;*
for my eyes have seen your salvation,
*   which you have prepared in the presence of all peoples,*
a light for revelation to the Gentiles
*   and for glory to your people Israel."*

Luke 2:29–32

Appendix A

Prayers for Catholics Struggling with Infertility

The Lord's Prayer

Our Father, who art in heaven, hallowed be thy name; thy kingdom come; thy will be done on earth as it is in heaven. Give us this day our daily bread, and forgive us our trespasses, as we forgive those who trespass against us, and lead us not into temptation, but deliver us from evil. Amen.

Hail Mary

Hail Mary, full of grace! The Lord is with you. Blessed are you among women, and blessed is the fruit of your womb, Jesus. Holy Mary, Mother of God, pray for us sinners, now and at the hour of our death. Amen.

The Salve Regina

Hail, holy Queen, Mother of mercy, our life, our sweetness, and our hope! To you we cry, poor banished children of

Eve; to you we send up our sighs, mourning and weeping in this valley of tears. Turn then, most gracious advocate, your eyes of mercy toward us, and after this our exile, show unto us the blessed fruit of your womb, Jesus. O clement, O loving, O sweet Virgin Mary.

The Memorare

Remember, O most gracious Virgin Mary, that never was it known that anyone who fled to your protection, implored your help, or sought your intercession was left unaided. Inspired by this confidence, I fly to you, O Virgin of virgins, my Mother. To you I come, before you I kneel sinful and sorrowful; O Mother of the Word Incarnate, despise not my petitions, but in your mercy, hear and answer me. Amen.

Memorare to Saint Joseph

Remember, O most chaste spouse of the Virgin Mary, that never was it known that anyone who implored your help and sought your intercession was left unassisted. Full of confidence in your powerful intercession, I fly to you and beg your protection. Despise not, O foster father of the Redeemer, my humble supplication, but in your goodness, hear and answer me. Amen.

Memorare to Saint Anne

Remember, good Saint Anne, whose name means grace and mercy, that never was it known that anyone who fled to your protection, implored your help, or sought your intercession, was left unaided. Inspired with this confidence, I come before you, sinful and sorrowful. Holy mother of the Immaculate Virgin Mary and loving grandmother of the

Savior, do not reject my appeal, but hear and answer me. Amen.

Prayer to the Holy Matriarchs and Saintly Women of the Bible

Righteous Sarah, bride of Abraham,
Holy Rebekah, bride of Isaac,
Blessed Rachel, bride of Jacob,
Godly bride of Manoah,
Faithful Hannah, bride of Elkanah,
Dear Saint Anne, bride of Joachim,
Sweet Elizabeth, bride of Zechariah,
All you holy matriarchs and saintly women,

God heard and answered your heartfelt prayers to deliver you from the sufferings of infertility. With humility and grief, I come before you, to beg for your holy intercession to our Lord on my behalf. Please beseech our Lord to heal my body and soul from the afflictions I bear and to place within my womb the gift of a child, one that I may raise to know and love the Lord our God, to serve him in this life, and to be with him forever in the world to come.

I implore and entreat you to ask that this favor be granted me, so that I may enjoy the spiritual benefits of the sacred vocation of motherhood, and one day come to join your holy company in heaven. Amen.

Prayer to Saint Gerard for Motherhood

O Good Saint Gerard, powerful intercessor before God, I come to ask your help. Beseech the Lord, the Giver of all life, to grant me the grace to conceive a child, if it be according to his plan. I hope to bear children who will be faith-filled disciples of Jesus, witnesses to his message of love, and heirs to the kingdom of heaven. Amen.

A Married Couple's Prayer to Saint Gerard

Saint Gerard, powerful intercessor before God, we come to ask your help. Beseech the Lord, the Giver of all life, to grant us the grace to bring new life into the world if it be according to his will. We desire and hope to be co-creators in God's plan of creation, to raise children who will be faith-filled disciples of Jesus, witnesses to his message of love, and heirs to the kingdom of heaven. Amen.

Prayer of Saint Gianna Beretta Molla

Jesus, I promise to submit myself to all that you permit to befall me, make me only know your will. My most sweet Jesus, infinitely merciful God, most tender Father of souls, and in a particular way of the most weak, most miserable, most infirm whom you carry with special tenderness in your divine arms, I come to you and ask you, through the love and merits of your Sacred Heart, the grace to understand and to always do your holy will, the grace to confide in you, the grace to rest securely through time and eternity in your loving divine arms.

Prayer at the Beginning of a New Cycle

Dear Lord, help us to begin again. Heal our sadness and give us hope. Awaken our faith and mend our hearts. Please God, let this be the cycle when we conceive our child. Deepen our love for each other and strengthen our marriage every time we come together as husband and wife. Let our love be fruitful and bring us the gift of a child. In our great longing, help us to remember that your will for our lives, not our will, brings us true happiness. Prepare our hearts to accept your will, whatever it may be. We make this prayer through Christ our Lord. Amen.

Prayer in a Time of Waiting

Dear Jesus, you know how desperately I want to be pregnant. As I near the end of this cycle, every twinge and minor ache I feel sends my hope soaring. It is too early to know if I am pregnant, and too late to change the outcome. Either I am pregnant or I am not. Only you know, Lord. My thoughts and energy are consumed by my intense desire. I try to convince myself that I am not pregnant to soften the potential disappointment, all the while desperately hoping that I am. I constantly tally the days from the beginning of this cycle, and count the months of potential pregnancy ahead. Help me, Lord, to give my heart to you. Protect me from the heartache that may await me, and carry me through these next few days sheltered in your love, until I know if I am a mother or not. Amen.

Prayer in a Time of Disappointment

O Father, we are so sad! For days we hoped that the tests were wrong. But they weren't. I'm not pregnant. O God, please help us, for this is so hard. Wrap us in your love, heal our broken hearts, and console us with hope for the future. Amen.

Prayer to Get Through the Holidays

Lord, everywhere I look I see people who are happy. I wish I could be happy, but I don't feel that way right now. I have no child to be thankful for. I have no child to buy Christmas presents for or bake cookies with. I do not look forward to beginning a new year or having another birthday without a child. I don't enjoy being around people who are laughing and singing when I feel like crying. I can't even turn on the television or go shopping without being reminded of what I don't have. Help me get through these next few weeks, Lord. Help me to focus on what I do have, especially for the gift of your son, Jesus, our Savior. And I pray that by this time next year I may have the gift of a child. Amen.

Prayer to Gain Perspective

Lord, forgive me for losing perspective. I so easily slip into the emotional routine of thinking first of my own suffering and desires. My self-consumed thoughts have blinded my eyes to the needs of others. While I desperately want to be pregnant, some women right now are desperately wishing they were not pregnant, perhaps even considering abortion. Please stir their hearts with your love for them. Give them grace to entrust their children's futures to you, either by giving them the ability to parent their children, or by leading them to make an adoption plan. Even as I long for a child, so many children throughout the world have no parents to love them, but rather are abandoned or neglected. Please allow their lives to be forever touched by the love of a permanent family. Lord, please protect me from losing my sense of perspective, and continue to open my eyes every day to the needs of those around me. Amen.

Prayer to Do God's Will

O Lord, we wish we knew your will for our lives. We would love to plan for the future, but we can't. We desperately want to be parents and are not ready to accept the fact that we may never conceive. We've thought about adoption, but we aren't really sure about that either. We are terrified by the thought of never having a child (*or: another child*). Please let us know what you want us to do next. We are ready to follow you, Lord, but you are silent. We know that what you want for us is better than anything we could ever imagine, but we don't know what it is. Make your will known to us, Lord. Enlighten our minds with your light, and let our hearts rest in your peace. Keep us from doing anything that goes against your will for us, and bring to completion the plan you have for us. Keep us close to you, so that we can follow you into whatever future you will guide us to. We make this prayer through Christ our Lord. Amen.

Prayer of Parents after Miscarriage
(Adapted from *Book of Blessings* 292, 293)

Loving God, comfort our hearts and grant that through the prayers of Mary, who grieved by the cross of her Son, you may enlighten our faith, give hope to our hearts, and peace to our lives. Receive this life you created in love and comfort us in our time of loss. Lord, grant us mercy and comfort us with the hope that one day we will all live with you, with your Son Jesus Christ, and the Holy Spirit, for ever and ever. Amen.

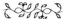

If you have already chosen possible names for the children you desire, you can pray to their patron saints to obtain for you the gift of a child. Information about many of the saints can be found online at www.catholic.org/saints/.

Appendix B

Biblical Men and Women Who Struggled with Infertility

For in the one Spirit we were all baptized into one body—Jews or Greeks, slaves or free—and we were all made to drink of one Spirit. . . . If one member suffers, all suffer together with it; if one member is honored, all rejoice together with it.

1 CORINTHIANS 12:13, 26

Throughout the world, many nomadic peoples make the desert their home. They do not navigate great distances in the desert alone, but travel in caravans. This ensures their protection and allows them to share the resources needed to survive. Together they travel in safety. Alone, they risk their lives.

When couples journey through infertility, they often feel as if they are completely alone. Fearful and isolated, they

struggle to find the resources they need for spiritual and emotional survival. They may not know that more than one in ten
couples experience infertility. They may not realize that when
they go to Mass, other people are also praying for the gift of a
child. Their feelings of isolation leave them emotionally and
spiritually vulnerable.

However, like nomadic peoples who navigate the desert
together, Catholics journey in a kind of spiritual caravan as
well. We call it the Communion of Saints. By virtue of our
Baptism, we are all spiritually connected to one another and
to the men and women who have gone before us into the
eternal life of heaven. We call them saints because we know
they are with God. Because we are all joined to Christ through
our faith, we are also joined to one another. The saints are
examples of holiness on whom we can model our lives and
through whose intercession we can rely for help. Just as we
ask our friends to pray for us, we can ask the saints to pray for
us as well.

Catholics who struggle with infertility journey through
their grief in this great company. Many holy men and women
throughout the ages have experienced infertility. Their stories
can be found in the Bible and in the Church's vast storehouse
of tradition—great stories of grief, hope, persistence, and
ultimate healing. Sometimes it can be painful to hear about
infertile couples who finally conceived and bore children,
because those of us who have not done so may feel left behind.
But sometimes it is encouraging to know that many years of
infertility can be overcome. The following stories taken from
the Bible can bring hope and offer you the company of holy
men and women who know exactly what you are going
through.

Abraham and Sarah (Genesis 15–21)

In the desert God promised Abraham, whose wife Sarah could not bear children, descendants as numerous as the sands of the earth and the stars of the sky (see Gen 15). After years of infertility, desperate for a child, they used Sarah's maidservant Hagar as a surrogate. Yet God continued to repeat his promise that Abraham and Sarah would conceive a child together. Abraham finally laughed in response, saying to himself, "Can a child be born to a man who is a hundred years old? Can Sarah, who is ninety years old, bear a child?" (Gen 17:17). Finally, after at least seventy years of infertility, well after Sarah had entered menopause, God fulfilled his promise. Sarah became pregnant and gave birth to Isaac. The impossible became possible, and it happened "at the time of which God had spoken to him" (Gen 21:2). God used this infertile couple, exceedingly advanced in years, to bring into existence countless generations of descendents who would become the Israelites, our ancestors in faith. The Gospel according to Saint Matthew and Saint Luke both give an account of the genealogy of Jesus, in which Isaac appears, the son of Abraham and Sarah.

Isaac and Rebekah (Genesis 24–25)

When he was forty years old, Isaac married Rebekah, and their marriage began the same way his parents' marriage did, with infertility. The Bible tells us that Rebekah was sterile. This couple was supposed to carry on the covenant that God had established with Abraham and make of their family a great and numerous people. How could that happen if Isaac and Rebekah could not conceive? Isaac prayed to God for his wife. Finally, Rebekah became pregnant with twins, though it seems she had a difficult pregnancy: "The children struggled together within her; and she said, 'If it is to be this way, why do I live?' So she went to inquire of the Lord" (Gen 25:22). After her ordeal, Rebekah delivered two healthy sons, Esau and Jacob.

Jacob and Rachel (Genesis 29–30)

Like their parents and grandparents, Rachel and Jacob could not conceive a child together. Infertility had become a family tradition. However, Jacob's other wife Leah, who happened to be Rachel's sister, was very fertile (it was customary at the time for a man to have more than one wife). Leah bore four sons to Jacob, while Rachel had none. Rachel was so jealous of her sister that she said to her husband, "Give me children, or I shall die!" (Gen 30:1). Like Sarah, Rachel gave her maidservant to her husband in order to have children with him through a surrogate. Rachel adopted the two sons her maidservant bore and so became a mother. Finally, after enduring years of infertility and intense suffering from her sister, the Bible says, "Then God remembered Rachel, and God heeded her and opened her womb. She conceived and bore a son, and said, "God has taken away my reproach; and she named him Joseph" (Gen 30:22–23). Rachel would later become pregnant again, but she died as she gave birth to her son Benjamin (Gen 35:18).

Manoah and His Wife (Judges 13)

A man named Manoah and his wife, whom the Bible does not name, were married while the Israelites were under the dominion of the Philistine people. She was barren, but an angel of the Lord appeared to her and promised her and

Manoah a son. They became the parents of Samson, who later delivered the Israelites from the power of the Philistines.

Elkanah and Hannah (1 Samuel 1:1–28)

Next the Bible brings us to Elkanah and Hannah. Elkanah loved his wife, "though the Lord had closed her womb. . . . She was deeply distressed and prayed to the Lord, and wept bitterly. She made this vow: 'O Lord of hosts, if only you will look on the misery of your servant, and remember me, and not forget your servant, but will give to your servant a male child, then I will set him before you as a nazirite until the day of his death. He shall drink neither wine nor intoxicants, and no razor shall touch his head'" (1 Sam 1:5, 10–11). God heard Hannah's prayer, and she conceived and bore Elkanah a son. They named him Samuel, and he became a great prophet.

Zechariah and Elizabeth (Luke 1:5–25)

Finally the Bible brings us to the story of Elizabeth and Zechariah. They were barren and advanced in years when the angel Gabriel appeared to Zechariah in the Temple to announce that he and Elizabeth would conceive and have a son. Zechariah did not believe Gabriel because he and his wife were so old. In punishment for his lack of faith, Zechariah lost his voice. He returned home and conceived a child with his wife. When Elizabeth discovered she was pregnant she exclaimed, "This is what the Lord has done for me when he looked favorably on me and took away the disgrace I have endured among my people" (Lk 1:25). Zechariah could not talk to her until after their baby was born. They named their son John, whom we now know as Saint John the Baptist.

Joachim and Anne

Though their story does not appear in the Bible, we learn from Catholic tradition that Anne and Joachim were also infertile. They were married for many years before an angel appeared to them, announcing God's promise of a child. They conceived and bore a daughter, whom they named Mary. Like Hannah, they dedicated their child to the Lord's service and raised her in a holy manner. Mary was betrothed to a man named Joseph, and though she remained a virgin, she became the mother of Jesus.

The Journey of Infertility

We will never meet a couple who struggled with infertility as long as Abraham and Sarah did. Poor Rebekah finally received what she so desperately wanted, only to suffer through a difficult pregnancy. How awful Rachel must have felt to witness her sister's seven pregnancies while she was infertile for so long. All of these Biblical figures had very unique and difficult journeys through infertility, yet God chose to use these three infertile couples for his great purpose. They became the ancestors of the Israelites, who later in history became known as the Jewish people. It is from these great matriarchs and patriarchs that Jesus himself can trace his ancestry.

Wouldn't it be wonderful to receive a clear message from God as did Manoah's wife, Zechariah, and Anne and Joachim? Surely many of us have tried to bargain with God in exchange for a child as Hannah did. The Blessed Mother, already with child, visited Elizabeth while she was pregnant. How wonderful it must have been for Elizabeth to share her long-awaited pregnancy with her young cousin.

All these couples eventually conceived and bore healthy children. Sadly, that may not be the case for all of us. However, these stories of strength, hope, and perseverance would not be diminished if these couples had never become parents. Their experience of infertility is not lessened because they later had a child, and perhaps it can give us hope. They can pray for us in the presence of God in heaven like no one else can, knowing our struggles because they shared them during their lifetimes.

One last group of people we meet in the Bible can tell us more about the desert. Throughout the Book of Exodus, we learn of how God led the people of Israel out of slavery in Egypt. God led them on a fateful journey to freedom in the Promised Land. But God did not lead them on a direct path. They spent forty years wandering lost in the desert, fearing they would die of hunger and thirst. In the desert they were stripped of everything that they had. In this punishing environment they realized their own weaknesses, and they were forced to acknowledge their daily dependence on God for everything they needed. God gave them food to eat and water to drink. Many of them would have preferred to leave the desert and return to slavery in Egypt. But it was because they were in the desert, vulnerable and broken, that they realized who they truly were before God. In the desert God revealed himself to them as their God, and they became his people. He made a new covenant with them and gave them his law. He revealed himself to Moses on his holy mountain, and Moses saw God face to face. God dwelt among his people in the desert.

The desert of the Israelites is our desert, for through our infertility God can accomplish his will for our lives. Here in the desert we can acknowledge our brokenness and dependence on God for our every need. In our vulnerability, God is inviting us to allow him to be our God, so that we may become his followers. Like the Israelites, most of us would prefer not to be in this desert. But if we can turn our lives over to God and allow him to lead us through the desert, we too will encounter his love and mercy. And eventually, if we keep following him, he will lead us to the land where the desert ends.

Appendix C

Patron Saints for Couples

Patron Saints to Protect against Infertility

Saint Agatha of Sicily
Saint Anne
Saint Anthony of Padua
Saint Casilda of Toledo
Saint Felicity of Rome
Saint Fiacre
Saint Giles

Saint Henry II
Saint Margaret of Antioch
Saint Medard
Saint Philomena
Saint Rita of Cascia
Saint Theobald Roggeri

Patron Saints to Protect against Miscarriage

Saint Catherine of Siena
Saint Catherine of Sweden

Patron Saints of Unborn Children

Saint Gerard Majella
Saint Joseph

Saint Gianna Beretta Molla

Patron Saints of Adopted Children

Saint Clotilde   Saint William of Rochester
Saint Thomas More

Patron Saints of Childless People

Saint Anne Line   Saint Henry II
Saint Catherine of Genoa   Saint Julian the Hospitaller
Saint Gummarus

Patron Saints of Fathers

Saint Joachim
Saint Joseph

Patron Saints of Mothers

Saint Anne   Saint Monica
Saint Gerard Majella   Saint Gianna Beretta Molla

Appendix D

Additional Resources

Church Documents

Catechism of the Catholic Church. United States Catholic Conference, Inc. Libreria Editrice Vaticana, 1994.

Dignitas Personae (Instruction on Certain Bioethical Questions). Congregation for the Doctrine of the Faith, 2008.

Donum Vitae (Instruction on Respect for Human Life in Its Origin and on the Dignity of Procreation). Congregation for the Doctrine of the Faith, 1987.

Evangelium Vitae (The Gospel of Life). Pope John Paul II, 1995.

Familiaris Consortio (Apostolic Exhortation on the Role of the Christian Family in the Modern World). Pope John Paul II, 1981.

Humane Vitae (Encyclical on the Regulation of Birth). Pope Paul VI, 1968.

Life-Giving Love in an Age of Technology. United States Conference of Catholic Bishops, 2009.

Night Prayer: From the Liturgy of the Hours. Washington, DC: United States Conference of Catholic Bishops, 1996.

The Truth and Meaning of Human Sexuality: Guidelines for Education within the Family. The Pontifical Council for the Family, 1995.

Books, Magazines, and Articles

Adoptive Families is a bimonthly magazine published by New Hope Media. Call 1–800–372–3300 for subscription information.

Alvaré, Helen. "Assisted Reproductive Technology and the Family." Respect Life Program, United States Conference of Catholic Bishops, 2007. Link can be found at: http://www.usccb.org/issues-and-action/human-life-and-dignity/reproductive-technology/.

Anderson, Marie, M.D., FACOG, and John Bruchalski, M.D. "Assisted Reproductive Technologies Are Anti-Woman." Respect Life Program, United States Conference of Catholic Bishops, 2004. Link can be found at: http://www.usccb.org/issues-and-action/human-life-and-dignity/reproductive-technology/.

Billings, Evelyn, and Ann Westmore. *The Billings Method: Controlling Fertility without Drugs or Devices*. Niagara Falls: Life Cycle Books, 2000.

Haas, John M., PhD, STL. "Begotten Not Made: A Catholic View of Reproductive Technology." Respect Life Program, United States Conference of Catholic Bishops, 1998. Link can be found at: http://www.usccb.org/issues-and-action/human-life-and-dignity/reproductive-technology/.

Hilgers, Thomas W., MD. *The NaProTechnology Revolution: Unleashing the Power in a Woman's Cycle*. New York: Beaufort Books, 2010.

Kippley, John and Sheila. *Natural Family Planning: The Complete Approach*. Raleigh, NC: Lulu Publishers, 2009.

May, William E. *Catholic Bioethics and the Gift of Human Life*. Huntington, IN: Our Sunday Visitor Books, 2000.

Packard, Jean Blair, ed. *In Their Own Words: Women Healed*. Omaha: Pope Paul VI Institute Press, 2004.

Shannon, Marilyn M. *Fertility, Cycles and Nutrition, 4th ed*. Cincinnati: Couple to Couple League, 2009.

West, Christopher. *Good News about Sex and Marriage: Answers to Your Honest Questions about Catholic Teaching*. Ann Arbor, MI: Servant Publications, 2000.

Wolfe, Jaymie Stuart. *The Call to Adoption: Becoming Your Child's Family*. Boston: Pauline Books & Media, 2005.

Finding a Doctor

To find a doctor in your area who is trained in NaPro-TECHNOLOGY, visit the Web site of Fertility*Care* Centers of America at www.fertilitycare.org and click on your state or region under "Find a Medical Consultant."

Internet

The National Center for Women's Health, associated with the Pope Paul VI Institute, is aligned with the Catholic Church's teachings on human reproduction and is one of the most successful infertility programs in the United States. The following Web sites are dedicated to different aspects of the mission of the Pope Paul VI Institute and are very helpful resources for couples struggling with infertility.

Pope Paul VI Institute for the Study of Human Reproduction	www.popepaulvi.com
Dr. Hilger's Personal Web site	www.drhilgers.com
NaProTECHNOLOGY	www.naprotechnology.com
The American Academy of FertilityCare Professionals	www.aafcp.org
FertilityCare Centers of America	www.fertilitycare.org
National Catholic Bioethics Center	www.ncbcenter.org
United States Conference of Catholic Bishops' Secretariat for Pro-Life Activities	www.usccb.org/prolife

Tate and Lottie Hilgefort provide support to couples who are struggling with infertility through their Web site, one-on-one contact, and support groups. Their site compiles a wealth of information on Catholic bioethics that is easy to understand and navigate. They also provide links to Catholic bloggers who are going through infertility. I wish the site had existed when my husband and I were going through infertility. www.catholicinfertility.org

Catholic Infertility Blogs

There are so many Catholics who have gone through infertility who share their experiences by blogging. Here are a few to get you started. The last blog listed is maintained by A. S., the woman who shared her story at the beginning of Chapter 4.

allyouwhohope.blogspot.com/
andnotbysight.blogspot.com/

frustrationstation-jellybelly.blogspot.com/
lavishedwithlemons.blogspot.com/
simone-perseverance.blogspot.com/
thiscrossiembrace.blogspot.com/

Adoption Web sites

www.adoption.com
www.catholic.adoption.com
www.catholiccharitiesusa.org/

You can find your local Catholic Charities office by going to the above Web site and clicking on "Get Help" to find your state. All the Catholic Charities offices in your state will be listed, and you can search their Web sites for information about adoption.

Fertility Awareness Organizations

Creighton Model FertilityCare System: www.creighton model.com

The Billings Ovulation Method: www.woomb.org

The Couple to Couple League International (Sympto-thermal method): www.ccli.org

Healing after Abortion

Project Rachel Information www.hopeafterabortion.com

Rachel's Vineyard Ministries www.rachelsvineyard.org.

Notes

Foreword

1. Joseph B. Stanford, MD, et. al., "Outcomes from Treatment of Infertility with Natural Procreative Technology in an Irish General Practice," *Journal of the American Board of Family Medicine* 21, no. 5 (Sept.–Oct. 2008): 375–384, http://www.jabfm.org/cgi/content/abstract/21/5/375.

2. Dr. Paul A. Carpentier, MD, is President of the American Academy of FertilityCare Professionals. He is a Certified FertilityCare Medical Consultant practicing in Gardner, Massachusetts, and he is Vice President of the Worcester Guild of the Catholic Medical Association. He was one of the first family physicians trained by Dr. Hilgers at the Pope Paul VI Institute for the Study of Human Reproduction in 1988. His office is named In His Image Family Medicine.

Chapter 1

1. Cf. Patricia Irwin Johnston, *Adopting after Infertility* (Indianapolis, IN: Perspectives Press, 1992).

2. Many women who adopt are able to nurse their children, but it may be difficult. For more information on this topic, see: Elizabeth Hormann. *Breastfeeding an Adopted Baby and Relactation* (New York: La Leche League International, 2007).

3. The psalm at the end of each chapter is selected from Night Prayer of the Divine Office, the daily liturgical prayer of the Church throughout the world. During our struggle with infertility, my husband and I found these prayers extremely helpful each night, as we were often unable to find our own words to pray. The psalms are poetic prayers that speak to God from

the depths of the human spirit. The psalms chosen for Night Prayer are particularly appropriate in tone for couples dealing with infertility and of unsurpassed spiritual and emotional value. They are available in an easy-to-use format in *Night Prayer From the Liturgy of the Hours*.

Chapter 3

1. Chapters 3 and 4 contain a thorough discussion of the moral principles involved in making decisions about the medical treatment of infertility, including artificial insemination, most often performed as Intra-Uterine Insemination (IUI).

2. If you do not know how to identify the fertile time in your cycle, Natural Family Planning (NFP) will help you tremendously. NFP is a natural method of identifying the time during the woman's cycle when she is fertile so that a couple may choose to postpone or achieve pregnancy. It is a morally acceptable and highly effective alternative to contraception, and it has helped innumerable people conceive. It also gives you valuable information about what is going on in your body and what may be going wrong, information that an over-the-counter ovulation predictor kit cannot give you.

3. R. P. Dickey, S. N. Taylor, P. H. Rye, et al., "Infertility Is a Symptom Not a Disease," *Fertility and Sterility* 74, no. 2 (2000): 398.

4. L. Lerner-Geva, J. Rabinovici, B. Lunenfeld, "Ovarian stimulation: Is there a long-term risk for ovarian, breast, and endometrial cancer?" *Women's Health* 6, no. 6 (Nov. 2010): 831–9.

J. Schneider, "Fatal colon cancer in a young egg donor: a physician mother's call for follow-up and research on the long-term risks of ovarian stimulation," *Fertil Steril* 90, no. 5 (Nov. 2008): 2016. e1-5. Epub (Mar. 2008).

L. Brinton, "Long-term effects of ovulation-stimulating drugs on cancer risk," *Reprod Biomed Online*, 15, no. 1 (Jul. 2007): 38–44.

5. "Ovarian Hyperstimulation Syndrome," *A.D.A.M. Medical Encyclopedia*. Reviewed by L. J. Vorvick, S. Storck, and D. Zieve on July 27, 2009.

6. Marie Anderson, MD, FACOG, and John Bruchalski, MD, "Assisted Reproductive Technologies Are Anti-Woman," Respect Life Program, United States Conference of Catholic Bishops (2004).

7. Stephanie Saul, "Birth of Octuplets Puts Focus on Fertility Clinics," *New York Times* (Feb. 11, 2009).

8. Ibid.

9. Joanna Perlman, "Is This Any Way to Have a Baby?" *O, The Oprah Magazine* (Feb. 1, 2004): 190.

10. See K. Riggan, "G12 Country Regulations of Assisted Reproductive Technologies," *Dignitas* 16 no. 4 (Winter 2009): 6–7. In Canada in 2004 the *Assisted Human Reproduction Act* established the regulation of certain aspects of the use of ART, set forth certain principles on its use, and created a regulatory body that oversees the enforcement of this legislation.

11. Pope Paul VI Institute for the Study of Human Reproduction, www.naprotechnology.com.

12. Ibid.

13. Over 99 percent of these cycles were IVF. See the 2009 National Summary Assisted Reproductive Technology (ART) Report published by the CDC online at http://apps.nccd.cdc.gov/art/Apps/NationalSummary Report.aspx.

14. T. W. Hilgers, *The Medical and Surgical Practice of* NaPro-TECHNOLOGY (Omaha, NE: Pope Paul VI Institute Press, 2004). Results vary based on the cause of infertility.

15. Pope Leo XIII, *On Christian Marriage*, no. 19.

16. See Ephesians 5:22–33.

17. *Donum Vitae*, Introduction, 3.

18. I highly recommend this book to Catholics who are unfamiliar with our faith's teachings on marriage and sexuality. For more information, see Appendix C.

19. For more on this topic, see: Erika Bachiochi, ed., *Women, Sex, and the Church: A Case for Catholic Teaching* (Boston: Pauline Books & Media, 2010).

20. *Dignitas Personae*, 12.

21. Ibid., 9.

22. *Donum Vitae*, II, A, 1.

23. *Dignitas Personae*, 12.

24. Ibid., 14.

Chapter 4

1. The Web sites for these different methods of NFP are listed in Appendix C under the heading "Fertility Awareness Organizations." There are also a number of books listed in this appendix that cover each of these methods in detail.

2. For a list of these fertility awareness organizations, see Appendix C.

3. You can access a database of doctors who are trained in NaProTECHNOLOGY online at www.fertilitycare.org by clicking on your state or region under "Find a Medical Consultant." The following was excerpted from http://www.popepaulvi.com/ncfwh-evaltreat.htm on

January 27, 2012: "The Pope Paul VI Institute Infertility Program, one of the few that exists in the United States, is a disease-based approach which recognizes that 'all infertility (or other reproductive problems) are caused by some type of organic or functional disease process.' Unlike the current medical approach, which typically involves limited evaluation, patients at the Pope Paul VI Institute will receive a complete evaluation and a sound explanation as to why they are having problems achieving or maintaining a pregnancy. The organic or functional causes of infertility can be relatively easily diagnosed and treated. . . . By identifying and treating the underlying diseases that cause infertility, the Institute harnesses the body's ability to work more effectively as opposed to 'driving' the reproductive system, 'pushing' the system, or trying to 'replace' the system. The effectiveness of the program varies depending upon the type of disease that occurs. In some cases, the Institute's effectiveness is greater than 80 percent in assisting a couple to successfully achieve a pregnancy. In many common infertility problems, the success rate will be 50 to 75 percent. In some more uncommon infertility problems, the success rate will be lower than that but almost always higher than the rates expected from programs driven by the artificial reproductive technologies (in vitro fertilization, artificial insemination, etc.). While the infertility program of the Pope Paul VI Institute is one of the most successful in the United States, a pregnancy can never be guaranteed."

4. Apex Medical Technologies manufactures a seminal fluid collection kit called Hy-gene Seminal Fluid Collection Kit. It is available in bulk cases for doctors to purchase online at www.apexfertility.com/hygene1.htm. You can call them at 1-800-345-3208 to request a free sample, or you can order them for individual use through ZDL, Inc at www.zdlinc.com/zdl_hygenekit.html.

5. You can call them at 402-390-6600 or visit them online at www.popepaulvi.com. There is more information on the Pope Paul VI Institute in Appendix C.

6. P. M. Zavos, "Characteristics of human ejaculates collected via masturbation and a new Silastic seminal fluid collection device," *Fertil Steril* 43 (1985): 491.

P. M. Zavos, "Seminal parameters of ejaculates collected from oligospermic and normospermic patients via masturbation and at intercourse with the use of a Silastic seminal fluid collection device," *Fertil Steril* 44 (1985): 517.

D. J. Mehan, M. J. Chehval, "A clinical evaluation of a new Silastic seminal fluid collection device," *Fertil Steril* 28 (1977): 689.

P. M. Zavos, "Comparison of two devices for semen collection during intercourse," *J of Andrology* 10 (1989): 82.

7. "Smoking and Infertility," Patient's Fact Sheet, American Society for Reproductive Medicine, www.asrm.org/uploadedFiles/ASRM_Content/Resources/Patient_Resources/Fact_Sheets_and_Info_Booklets/smoking.pdf. Retrieved on 11/21/2010.

8. "Weight," American Society for Reproductive Medicine, www.asrm.org/topics/detail.aspx?id=1763. Retrieved on 11/21/2010.

9. "Highlights from the 66th Annual Meeting: Fat and Fertility in Men," Press Release, American Society for Reproductive Medicine (Oct. 25, 2010).

10. For more information on nutrition, supplements, and fertility, see: Shannon, *Fertility, Cycles & Nutrition, 4th ed.* Also, keeping the bedroom dark is very valuable for both helping infertility and preventing miscarriage. See DeFelice, Joy, R.N., B.S.N., P.H.N, The Effects of Light on the Menstrual Cycle: Also Infertility (Spokene, WA: Sacred Heart Medical Center, 2000).

11. "Stress and Infertility," Patient Fact Sheet, American Society for Reproductive Medicine, www.asrm.org/uploadedFiles/ASRM_Content/Resources/Patient_Resources/Fact_Sheets_and_Info_Booklets/Stress-Fact.pdf. Retrieved on 11/21/2010. In an occasional woman, acute stress (indicated by sweaty palms, increased heart rate, and heavy breathing) may cause hormonal shifts that result in delayed or skipped ovulation in a particular cycle. However, this is different from the underlying chronic stress that often accompanies infertility. The latter type of stress has never been shown to be the cause of infertility.

12. There are a number of helpful prayers included in Appendix A.

13. A varicocele is an abnormal enlargement of the vein in the scrotum which results in a pooling of blood in that area of the blood vessel. This pooling of blood can raise the temperature in the scrotum just enough to create a suboptimal environment for sperm production, often leading to male infertility. Recent research shows that over 90 percent of male infertility is caused by bilateral varicoceles, and the condition is almost always treatable with outpatient surgery.

14. See www.naprotechnology.com/surgical.htm.

15. Haas, "Begotten Not Made: A Catholic View of Reproductive Technology."

16. The guidelines that follow are based on the Church's teachings as articulated in *Donum Vitae* and *Dignitas Personae*. These documents are listed in Appendix B.

17. *Dignitas Personae*, 16.

18. Cf. *CCC*, nos. 2376–2377.

19. *Dignitas Personae*, 17.

20. *Donum Vitae*, I, 5.

21. Ibid., I, 6.

22. *Dignitas Personae*, 18.

23. Ibid., 15.

24. Ibid., 28.

25. For more Catholic resources on human cloning and other bioethical issues, see the National Catholic Bioethics Center Web site at www.ncbcenter.org. You can find resources listed by topic.

26. For more information about different theologian's moral evaluations of GIFT, see: John M. Hass, "Gift? No!" *Ethics and Medics*, Pope John Center, Braintree, MA, 18, no. 9 (Sept. 1993): 1–3; and Donald G. McCarthy, "Gift? Yes!" *Ethics and Medics*, Pope John Center, Braintree, MA, 18, no. 9 (Sept. 1993): 3–4.

27. *Donum Vitae*, II, B, 6.

28. David I. Hoffman, MD, et al., "Cryopreserved embryos in the United States and their availability for research," *Fertility and Sterility* 79, no. 5 (May 2003).

29. Jessica Lukawiecki, "Frozen in Limbo," *McGill Daily* (March 29, 2011) http://www.mcgilldaily.com/2011/03/frozen-in-limbo/.

30. Data retrieved from http://www.cdc.gov/ART/ART2006/section5.htm#f64 on 5/1/2010.

31. In paragraph 19, *Dignitas Personae* clearly states "The proposal that these embryos could be put at the disposal of infertile couples as a *treatment for infertility* is not ethically acceptable for the same reasons which make artificial heterologous procreation [use of donor sperm or eggs] illicit as well as any form of surrogate motherhood; this practice would also lead to other problems of a medical, psychological, and legal nature."

32. *Dignitas Personae*, 19.

33. USCCB. "Questions and Answers: The Instruction 'Dignitas Personae*: On Certain Bioethical Questions,'" (Dec. 9, 2008). Retrieved from http://www.usccb.org/comm/Dignitaspersonae/Q_and_A.pdf on 12/5/2009.

34. For a good discussion of both sides of the issue, see Richard Grebenc, "Frozen Embryo Disposition: The Catholic Discussion," http://duq.academia.edu/RichardGrebenc/Papers/601103/_Frozen_Embryo_Disposition_The_Catholic_Discussion_. See also "What Should We Do with the Frozen Embryos?" by Father Tadeusz Pacholczyk, PhD, http://www.catholiceducation.org/articles/medical_ethics/me0137.htm; "The Absurd Fate of Frozen Embryos: Interview with Law Professor Brian Scarnecchia," by Andrea Kirk Assaf, http://www.zenit.org/e-28463.

35. *Dignitas Personae*, 16.

36. *Donum Vitae*, Introduction, 1.

37. Ibid., II, B, 5.

38. Haas, "Begotten Not Made: A Catholic View of Reproductive Technology."

Chapter 5

1. *CCC*, no. 2373.

Chapter 6

1. See A. D. Domar, et. al., "The psychological impact of infertility: a comparison with patients with other medical conditions." *Journal of Psychosomatic Obstetrics and Gynaecology* 14 (1993): 45–52.

Chapter 7

1. If your life has been touched by the loss of a child through abortion, you are not alone. There is hope and healing available. Project Rachel is the Catholic Church's ministry of healing that reaches out to those who have suffered this traumatic loss. You can find more information online at http://www.hopeafterabortion.com. Rachel's Vineyard, a ministry of Priests for Life, offers weekend retreats to help those mourning the loss of a child through abortion. Their Web site is http://www.rachelsvineyard.org.

2. For information about STDs and infertility, see www.cdc.gov/std/infertility/default.htm. Both chlamydia and gonorrhea can cause infection in the uterus and fallopian tubes and can lead to pelvic inflammatory disease, which can result in infertility. These STDs can also cause complications during pregnancy. G.R. Huggins, V. E. Cullins, "Fertility after contraception or abortion," *Fertil Steril* 54, no. 4 (Oct. 1990): 559–73.

3. For a thorough discussion of the relationship between abortion and infertility see Chapter 4: "Impact on Subsequent Pregnancies," and Chapter 5: "Future Fertility" in Elizabeth Ring-Cassidy and Ian Gentles *Women's Health after Abortion*, 2nd Edition (Toronto: deVeber Institute, 2003).

4. G. R. Huggins, V. E. Cullins, "Fertility after contraception or abortion," *Fertil Steril* 54, no. 4 (Oct. 1990): 559–73.

5. Ibid.

Chapter 8

1. Chapters three and four explain why IVF is not an acceptable moral option.

2. We also share the company of many other men and women who know this desert of infertility well. The many matriarchs, patriarchs, and saints who have walked where we now stand are our companions. Their stories, recorded in the Bible and found in Appendix B, can be sources of hope and strength as we journey through the desert.

Chapter 9

1. Jewish law in the Old Testament did not actually provide for adoption, so I am using these biblical examples in a somewhat wide sense of the term.

2. The following information about the different ways to build a family through adoption is based on the most current information available as reported in "2010 Adoption Options," *Adoptive Families* (March/April 2010): 28–33.

3. See Michael Bohman, *Adopted Children and Their Families* (Stockholm, Sweden: Proprius, 1970).

4. This does not mean, however, that couples who are able to conceive may deliberately exclude children altogether from their marriage. Such an intention would invalidate their sacrament of marriage.

5. *CCC*, no. 1654.

6. Johnnette S. Benkovic, *Full of Grace: Women and the Abundant Life* (Cincinnati: Saint Anthony Messenger Press, 2004).

Chapter 10

1. A miscarriage is a pregnancy loss prior to viability, roughly twenty weeks. A stillbirth is a much later and rarer pregnancy loss, when the baby dies in utero any time from viability to full term.

2. *CCC*, no. 404.

3. Ibid., no. 310.

Chapter 11

1. *The Official Revised Baltimore Catechism Number One* (New York: William H. Sadlier, Inc., 1944), 2.

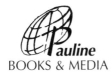

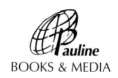

auline
BOOKS & MEDIA

The Daughters of St. Paul operate book and media centers at the following addresses. Visit, call or write the one nearest you today, or find us on the World Wide Web, www.pauline.org

CALIFORNIA
3908 Sepulveda Blvd, Culver City, CA 90230	310-397-8676
935 Brewster Avenue, Redwood City, CA 94063	650-369-4230
5945 Balboa Avenue, San Diego, CA 92111	858-565-9181

FLORIDA
145 S.W. 107th Avenue, Miami, FL 33174	305-559-6715

HAWAII
1143 Bishop Street, Honolulu, HI 96813	808-521-2731
Neighbor Islands call:	866-521-2731

ILLINOIS
172 North Michigan Avenue, Chicago, IL 60601	312-346-4228

LOUISIANA
4403 Veterans Memorial Blvd, Metairie, LA 70006	504-887-7631

MASSACHUSETTS
885 Providence Hwy, Dedham, MA 02026	781-326-5385

MISSOURI
9804 Watson Road, St. Louis, MO 63126	314-965-3512

NEW YORK
64 West 38th Street, New York, NY 10018	212-754-1110

PENNSYLVANIA
Philadelphia—relocating	215-676-9494

SOUTH CAROLINA
243 King Street, Charleston, SC 29401	843-577-0175

VIRGINIA
1025 King Street, Alexandria, VA 22314	703-549-3806

CANADA
3022 Dufferin Street, Toronto, ON M6B 3T5	416-781-9131

¡También somos su fuente para libros,
videos y música en español!